Mind *over Medicine*
can the mind *kill or cure*?

Robin Blake was born in Preston, Lancashire in 1948. He
read English at Cambridge and taught for six years in Suffolk,
London, Bulgaria and Turkey. In 1979 he joined Capital
Radio to make educational programmes. He later became
a features producer with a special interest in health and
medicine and was responsible for starting a weekly health
news programme, *Check Up*.

In addition to numerous documentary features on various
subjects, he has written and produced several plays for the
Independent Radio network. He now writes freelance and
lectures part-time in Radio at Goldsmiths College. With
Eleanor Stephens he is author of the psychological study
Compulsion (1987).

Robin Blake is married with two sons and lives in North
London.

Robin Blake

MIND over MEDICINE
can the mind kill or cure?

Pan Original
Pan Books
London and Sydney

First published 1987 by Pan Books Ltd
Cavaye Place, London SW10 9PG
9 8 7 6 5 4 3 2 1
© Robin Blake 1987
ISBN 0 330 29536 5

Phototypeset by
Input Typesetting Ltd, London SW19 8DR
Printed in Great Britain by Cox & Wyman Reading

For my parents, John and Beryl Blake

Contents

Acknowledgements

I am grateful for the assistance of the Institute of Noetic Science in San Francisco, the Pain Relief Foundation in Walton, Liverpool, the Psoriasis Association, the National Association for the Childless, the Bristol Cancer Help Centre, and the British Psychological Society.

Many individuals have given me their time, but I am particularly glad to acknowledge Dr Robert Seville, Dr Lopsang Rapgay of New Delhi and the healer Andrew Watson. In addition, my friends Dr Ben Lloyd and Dr Adam Timmis have provided not only intellectual stimulation but much practical help, whilst politely dissenting from many of my ideas.

Finally, I am more than indebted to another generous dissenter, Professor William Waugh, who read my manuscript and played Devil's Advocate.

Figure one is reproduced by permission of the British Library.

QALYS and quantities

I shall begin with an excursion forward in time. It is twenty years from now and I am nearly sixty years of age. My future self has become increasingly preoccupied with health, as the accumulated stress of three-quarters of a lifetime has begun to assert itself. Every year I am a little less hungry and a little more paunchy; deafer, but less tolerant of loud noise; more exhausted at night, but less likely to sleep night-long.

At this point, though, there is something new. Instead of feeling hungry in the morning I am nauseous, and have vague discomfort bordering on heartburn. For a week I suffer in silence. Then, one night, I throw up my supper and with it a quantity of blood. Now I am scared.

I go at once to the computer terminal under the stairs and dial into the District Health Authority's computer. I am asked to key in my symptoms. For a few moments the computer consults my personal medical file and the screen is blank. Then a message is flashed across it: 'PLEASE ATTEND H.M.U. AT ONCE'. It gives me a reference to quote.

That morning I call at the nearest Health Maintenance Unit. Once inside the consultation booth I make myself known to the terminal by keying in the reference code. On request, I stand in front of the body-scanner and subsequently answer a detailed questionnaire from the screen. I am then told to go home and rest until contacted.

Eventually, of course, I will see a doctor. But by then the preliminary computer-diagnosis will have been assessed in the light of my medical history, genetic profile and personal details. All the options in my case will thus be easily and painlessly determined; the doctor will merely have to resolve anomalies, if any, and offer me such treatment as the computer suggests.

This is an advanced socialized medical system and in deciding whether or not I should be offered free treatment, the computer makes use of the QALY. This stands for 'Quality Adjusted Life Year', a unit of account assigning a numerical value to the *quality* of any extra years of life which the treatment of a given patient with a given illness yields. To the cost-conscious, resources-starved medical service, the QALY is a beautiful invention. It is clean, precise and scrupulously fair – an administrator's dream, which enables all dilemmas about priorities in treatment to be reduced entirely to mathematics. You simply divide the cost of treatment by the number of QALYs, and you then have an exact prediction of the return society can expect to receive on its investment.

Thus – supposing I have, as I suspect, something seriously wrong with me – my chances of being treated free will depend on the diagnosis. A sixty-year-old with a perforated ulcer might have a quick operation and be rehabilitated in a few weeks, so in this case a cheap course of treatment returns plenty of QALYs. However, an advanced tumour would be a very different matter. Assuming that, in twenty years' time, stomach cancer still involves difficult treatment and a poor prognosis, then a much greater outlay will yield many fewer QALYs. So the probability is that, if my sixty-year-old time-travelling self has an ulcer, they treat it. If I am unlucky enough to have cancer, they reserve me a bed in the hospice.

Why does this fantasy feel so uncomfortable? After all, I receive prompt and efficient attention and am dealt with in an entirely democratic spirit. Yet what offends is the very coldness and inhumanity of this egalitarian treatment. The sick person who can be so comprehensively appraised by machines is reduced to no more than a machine. The free individual who can be crimped to fit the value-system represented by the QALY is no longer either free *or* an individual, but an abstraction, a statistical aggregate yoked to a few bytes of computer information.

My time-traveller's horror story is set two decades in the future, but its basic elements are already upon us. I first heard of London teaching hospitals using electronic research questionnaires with patients more than six years ago. The pressure on doctors' time – time which is increasingly expensive – is such that consultations are already being cut to the barest minimum; any further reduction can only mean computer assistance.

2

Meanwhile, electronic storage and retrieval of medical files is commonplace.

Computer diagnosis, too, is already with us in some fields: computerized axial tomography ('whole body scanning') is a diagnostic tool of unrivalled sophistication. Equally sophisticated is the diagnostic software of 'expert systems'. This is where the combined knowledge of distinguished experts is written into a program, so that probable diagnoses and alternatives can be arrived at. There is no doubt that such programming, still at a fairly primitive stage of development, will make great strides in the next decade.

But what of the QALY? Surely, that at least is Huxleyan make-believe. In fact, the QALY is the invention of economists at the Centre for Health Economics at the University of York, and is under serious discussion as a possible yardstick of economic efficiency in Britain's Health Service. It is taken sufficiently seriously to have been the subject of a seminar organized by the British Medical Association in 1986.

Medicine's use of reductionism – the process of breaking things up or fining them down until they appear in manageable units – is extensively criticized in what follows. Reductionism, when it goes too far, always ends up being ridiculous, and the logical extensions of computer diagnosis and the QALY threaten medicine with palpable absurdity. However, this does not mean I want to see all reductionist enquiry obliterated: that would be like trying to abolish left feet. Just as we have a left foot and a right foot, so we employ alternative ways of looking at the world – one which takes things to pieces, the *reductive*, and one which looks at wholes, the *integrative*. The alternatives complement each other and can normally claim equal validity, although on occasion one mode predominates. The trouble with modern medicine is that it has been exclusively left-footed whilst engaged in an activity – healing – which I would argue ought to favour the other foot.

Reductionism has undeniably achieved remarkable medical feats. Highlights include the development of the polio vaccine, the synthesis of hormones, the introduction of antibiotics, tissue-grafting (initially for burns) and the restoration of mobility by means of artificial limbs and limb-joints. Diseases which were formerly large-scale killers and have been neutralized or at least brought under control include leprosy, rickets,

3

syphilis, smallpox, TB, scurvy, yellow fever, typhus and enteric fever. Symptomatic treatments exist for many other major chronic diseases including schizophrenia, Parkinson's disease and diabetes. Effective treatments exist, too, for common minor conditions like herpes, enlarged prostate, short-sightedness and varicose veins. Almost everyone has had cause to be thankful for some of these techniques and only a fool would deny their worth.

Yet the worth must come into perspective and, as usual, that means examining the context. Contexts, of course, are relative matters and the relativity at the back of medicine is obvious – the patients. The successes of scientific medicine have been won in the teeth of an uncomfortable fact: patients are people, and people are all different.

For four decades governments in developed countries have been encouraged to build and maintain vast and cumbersome corporations through which to channel the production of national health. In Britain the contract goes almost exclusively to the nationalized Health Service, the largest employer in Europe except for the Red Army. The original object of the National Health Service can be described (only slightly satirically) as first ironing out inequalities in the population's health, then gradually whittling away all ill-health until at last the population consists entirely of rosy-cheeked individuals who will bound uncomplainingly through life before dying naturally at a ripe age. Any disease which does unfortunately occur can be quickly put in its place by a rational cure. Thus the hospitals were to be largely concerned with the relatively short-term treatment of serious illness, while GPs carried out such maintenance and minor repairs as would, from time to time, be necessary.

The vision has long ago been consigned to the realm of fantasy. First, the hospitals have become victims of superficial success. Undoubtedly they are very good at keeping people alive for rather longer than before, but extending life does not always amount to cure and more than half the beds in British hospitals are occupied by long-term chronic patients, most of them elderly. The majority of these can expect no cure, but must wait out their lives as more or less helpless dependants of the hospital. This, often referred to as the state of being 'institutionalized', is the very opposite of the efficiency and rapid through-put of the once-envisaged NHS hospital. It is the

4

dilemma presented by this vast and growing population of the institutionalized which tempts hard-pressed administrators to seek salvation in the QALY.

GPs bear an unexpectedly heavy load too. Routine health-maintenance, far from being a diminishing burden, steadily increases. In the 1970s, the number of men taking time off work because of illness increased by almost one–sixth and of women by no less than one-third. According to the British *General House-hold Survey*, there was in that decade a 45 per cent increase in the number of people reporting long-standing health problems. The existence of a wide variety of drugs means that the doctor can keep people functioning, but is frequently unable to touch the underlying problems.

Drugs are not, of course, intrinsically evil, though the way in which they are used can be very damaging. More neutrally, drugs usually act as a substitute – more or less adequate – for some substance which the body normally produces itself, but through a metabolic defect has failed to do so. A famous and effective example is insulin for diabetics. Yet insulin replace-ment does not confront the causes of the illness, it side-steps them – a pharmacological equivalent of spare-part surgery. The fact that the use of insulin is a life-saving intervention which can result in a reasonably normal life for the patient does not invalidate the point. The diabetic is not cured by insulin, but is chained to it even more inseparately than the one-legged man to his crutch.

Two out of five people go to the doctor with psychological problems, and in the last forty years these have been almost universally treated with drugs. Drug treatment is often used not because the medicine will do any good, but as an expression of helplessness. As one doctor put it:

A lot of these psychological conditions are really untreatable – brought about by social circumstances that you cannot change. I mean, one can't really solve social situations which have developed over years with a few hours of chat. It's pompous to think you can. You just uncover a mess that you can't clear up. You can't change these circumstances by giving pills either, but you can influence people to an extent by giving them faith in an anti-depressant. I think that's a good thing. But I'm a bit sceptical about the actual effects of these sorts of drugs.[1]

Unfortunately, the effect is often that the 'faith' which some patients find in these drugs is merely that of the addict, since it is now known that the most widely prescribed anti-depressants, the benzodiazapines – Valium, Librium, etc – often create dependency in people who use them for more than a few weeks.

The vision of socialized medicine was an impossible one, as we can now recognize, but all the consequences of that recognition have not yet filtered through. As patients and as politicians we continue to make extraordinary demands on medical services, fully supported by pharmaceutical companies and representatives of the professions for whom the medical *status quo* represents a good living. Thus any radical reshaping of the health service so as to reflect a new, more realistic appraisal of the role of medicine is seen as morally and politically 'impossible': medicine is too deeply embedded in our social structures. Even limited reform is portrayed as equivalent to dismantling the health services altogether. Cash limits or limited-list prescribing are seen as attacks on clinical freedom and on patients' lives. The push for more machinery, more specialization, more research money comes unremittingly from all quarters. To a very large extent, then, we have the health service we deserve.

The paradox is that today, as demands on medicine become greater, there is at the same time growing disillusion with it. The consensus which created Britain's monolithic National Health Service, a modern and model expression of medical orthodoxy, does perhaps still exist, but it is finally showing signs of coming apart. There is a growing crisis of faith not only in medicine's power to cure, but in its power to *explain*. In many ways the latter is the more damaging blow, because it involves a deeper level of credibility.

Take, for example, the phenomenon of *fatigue*. This is one of the most common of symptoms, yet is also a perfectly 'normal' state. What can science tell us about it? Muscle fatigue is to do with the by-products of muscle chemistry accumulating faster during hard work than the blood flow can remove them. It may also be a result of swelling caused by the seepage of fluids into the muscle tissue during work. The physical effect is to interfere with and restrict the action of nerve cells controlling the muscles. Thus far science takes us; it says little, however, about the links between muscle fatigue and the mental feeling of tiredness such as we all have at the end of the day, or at times of illness. The difference between healthy and unhealthy fatigue is unknown – indeed, this most common of nervous states is almost entirely a mystery. There is a physical effect: our reflexes are slow, our limbs feel heavy, our attention span is limited. But fatigue is more convincingly associated with purely mental than with physical phenomena. Boredom brings it on and it can be easily alleviated by mood-changing drugs such as alcohol or amphetamines. It comes in cycles and may be relieved by sleep. But sleep – undoubtedly a measurable physical state – is itself an almost wholly mysterious activity, with no known rationale. As one popular reference work on medicine says, 'Until more is known of sleep and the reasons for it, tiredness has to be defined as the need for sleep, and sleep as that which relieves tiredness'.[2] However, even this circularity – which itself is a scientific embarrassment – does not properly cover the experience of fatigue. Many people *wake up* tired; many exhausted people suffer insomnia. Fatigue, in fact, is a mental phenomenon whose association with physical states is almost wholly unexplained.

Reductionist research has provided some clues to the states of sleep and fatigue, but I cannot see that it will ever explain them. These are *holistic* phenomena, involving the entire mind-body continuum. However, reductionist biology by definition does not deal at this level, since the mind-body cannot be isolated to fulfil experimental conditions. Yet why should fatigue and sleep be any different from other biological phenomena? Life is about systems and about inter-action between systems – physical, mental and spiritual – and understanding cannot be reached by a reductionist viewpoint whose only overall picture is of a sack filled with soft machinery. By looking at smaller and smaller particles of being, mechanical biologists move steadily further from the idea of the *whole* and so, although they produce much knowledge and many medical techniques, in a sense they are always working against the grain of nature.

Mind, as the late Gregory Bateson argued so compellingly in his *Mind and Nature*[3], is by definition involved in every biological system. The mollusc mind may be rudimentary, but it exists and the more highly organized systems of human biology develop with a more complex mind. This includes not only consciousness but the shadowy area of the unconscious. But mind is not a *part* of the body; it is an integrative principle of the *whole*. Therefore it is involved in all health and all illness and it comprehends our bodies to an extent which reductionism, operating from the *outside* as it were, has never accepted.

Reductionist medicine still almost universally controls our significant agencies of healing. Yet it is increasingly on the defensive, perhaps even in the very first stages of decline. This book is intended in a very small way to grease its path. My fundamental argument is that, in illness, too much importance must not be placed on our interchangeable mechanical parts, although it is on the basis of these alone that scientific doctors build their universal hypotheses. On the contrary, the important factors in healing are those which define us as integrated, whole and individual. We are all interconnected with each other, of course; but each is also quite unique. Our uniqueness – which can become rather a strange idea in a reductionist world – is expressed first of all in the mental and the spiritual aspects of our nature. But since mind and spirit do quite literally permeate our physical lives – our organs and connective tissue no less than our style of dress and our daily activities – then if we wish to achieve real understanding of organic illness, we must start by placing our habitual dependence on reductionist medicine *beneath* a new awareness of the role of the mind.

Chapter 1

Heart and harmony

'Every disease is a musical problem; every
cure a musical solution'
Novalis

'The best doctors are like beautiful violinists'
– *Svyataslov Fyodorov (Soviet eye-surgeon)*

*T*he heart is regarded, by many who think of the body in this way, as the supreme mechanical, automated component. Our life depends on its independence, consistency, strength and persistence in performing its tasks within strict specifications and under a wide variety of circumstances. Surely this is the greatest triumph of pre-programmed bio-mechanics?

Well, yes, but there is much more to it than that. Above all the body's organs, the heart has *meaning*, a place in our mental universe which is quite as significant as its bodily function. In this chapter I shall examine both aspects of what, since the earliest times, has been seen as our central organ.

The objective heart

Even viewed dispassionately as a hunk of matter, this mechanical paragon reveals many different sides to itself. Fundamental is its character as one big muscle which, like all muscles, is threaded by a network of blood vessels supplied with nutrients by the coronary arteries. It contains four chambers which are linked, in pairs, by one-way valves.

Small organisms with simple blood circulation have no need of such a muscle, but the heart's evolution – out of a knot of muscular fibre surrounding a single section of the primitive central blood vessel – accompanied and made possible the appearance of more complex forms of life. Of these, humanity is the prize exhibit.

The image of the heart as a pump is popular but incorrect. It is *two* pumps: one, on the right side, driving the blood from the veins of the body into the lungs to pick up oxygen; the other, on the left, pushing the oxygenated blood – as it returns from the lungs – into the arteries and round the body. Thomas Ewbank, a nineteenth-century historian and author of *Hydraulic and other Machines for Raising Water*, made so bold as to reduce the human body to these functions:

> Every human being may be considered as, nay is, a living pump. His body is wholly made up of it, of the tubes belonging to it, and the liquid moved by it – with such additions as are required to communicate the necessary motion and protect it from injury.

Ewbank tells us that the working of the pump is the 'unerring criterion' used to determine the state of a person's health 'or, as an engineer would say, the number of its strokes per minute is the proof of its state, whether in good or bad working order.' And he allows himself a moment of astonishment at the machine's technical excellence:

> Formed of materials so easily injured, and connected with tubes of the most delicate texture, whose ramifications are too complex to be traced, their numbers too great to be counted, and many of them too minute to be perceived, and the orifices all furnished with elaborate valves; that such complicated machinery should continue incessantly in motion for sixty, eighty, and a hundred years .... is as inexplicable and mysterious as the power that impels it.[1]

Certainly any letter of testimony written to commend this piece of engineering would be impressive. Firstly, it possesses an unusual degree of autonomy. Breathing, too, is thought of as an 'autonomous' system, in that it can continue when we are asleep or unconscious. But the muscles of breathing cannot work without some minimal input from the brain, known as the 'neurogenic drive'. The heart is independent even of neurogenic drive. This explains why people who are considered 'brain-dead' can still be kept going on a respirator. As long as the heart has blood that contains oxygen, it will pump that blood.

Secondly, its endurance is extraordinary. The normal heart is the body's most efficient muscle in the use of energy, yet the power it expends in one day would be sufficient to lift a ton weight. On average, it contracts and relaxes forty million times a year and, in each and every hour of that year, pumps between seventy and a hundred gallons of blood. It never takes a holiday, not even a few minutes off, but must continue to work through all but the most serious disruptions. This means that the injured heart needs tremendous powers of self-repair, to be exercised while it still goes on working.

Thirdly, the heart is adaptable. It adjusts its work-rate incessantly (if necessary, it can double it) to cater for the body's energy needs. It must also adapt to atmospheric pressure. The further away you are from the earth's centre, the lower the pressure of oxygen in the lungs and the harder the heart must work if the blood is to retrieve enough of it. Short-term adjustment, abolishing the symptoms of mountain sickness, starts within a few hours; adjustment in the hearts of long-term emigrants to a higher (or lower) altitude happens over weeks and months. So if its owner is inclined to take up mountaineering, or living in Tibet, or on the ocean bed in a bathysphere, his willing slave the heart follows.

Fourthly, the heart is virtually irreplaceable. There are coronary robots capable of taking over the heart function during cardiac surgery, but these are over-sized and can only be temporary stand-ins. Certain of the heart's functions can be replaced by artificial components, such as the electronic pacemaker or even a prosthetic valve. But on the very day I write this the newspapers are reporting the death of William Schroeder, twenty months after the operation to insert an artificial aluminium and plastic heart inside his chest. Several people have so far been fitted experimentally with the device at the Humana Heart Institute at Louisville, Kentucky, with Schroeder the longest survivor. But it cannot be said that his QALYs were particularly good ones. He suffered four strokes after the operation, and was confused and unable to speak during his last eight months. Animals have survived longer with artificial hearts, but a portable blood-pump for humans which matches

11

the compactness. subtlety and durability of the real thing is still a long way away.

William Schroeder was one of a small elite of heart patients chosen to go over the top in the furtherance of replacement surgery. Others have been Philip Blaiburg (the first heart transplant patient) and 'Baby Rae' who, in California in 1985, received the heart of a baboon. The deaths of these pioneers, when they inevitably occur, are the tip of a vast iceberg of heart patients who succumb every year to a disease which has placed most of them far beyond the range and resources of medical science.

The heart is most vulnerable in its personal energy supply. If the arteries which circulate oxygenated blood through it become narrowed (atherosclerosis) and then blocked (coronary thrombosis), you have a sudden crisis in which the muscle fibres are starved of oxygen and damaged. The resulting pain is often described as a constricting pain (*angina pectoris*) in a band across the chest. If the heart's pumping action is weakened, breathlessness and fatigue follow. The pumping action can also be affected if the valves – which ensure uni-directional blood flow through the heart – are damaged.

Any shortfall in the heart's blood supply immediately triggers a process of compensation. The total volume of blood increases as the kidneys scale down the amount of fluid they extract from it – with the aim, perhaps, of boosting the damaged heart's output. But longer-term effects of an inefficient heart follow: *build-up* of fluid outside the blood vessels, especially in the legs (known as oedema), faster heartbeat and pulse, and perhaps an irregular ryhthm (fibrillation). Sensing the heart's impairment, the failing cardiovascular system gradually withdraws service from the body's outlying parts, starting with the legs (and causing the oedema). The last part to be abandoned is the brain. Unconsciousness and death follow if the heart stops beating. These are the objective facts about the heart's ills.

The subjective heart

The heart is the perfect servant, playing an omnicompetent Jeeves opposite the Bertie Wooster that is in each of us. The peerlessness of Jeeves is that, though he has a superb *mind* of his own, he has no *will*. His loyalty to the feckless, factuous Wooster comes from the recognition that they are wound and bound together by common threads of fate and dependency. The failure of one leads to the downfall of the other. Neither Jeeves nor the heart can afford to go their own way, nor even to have private desires. They may decisively influence events but they do not dictate them – except by a form of blackmail, such as when Jeeves threatens Wooster with his notice, of which the cardiac equivalent is perhaps *angina pectoris*.

Yet our dependence is more than a mechanical requirement. Culturally, humanity is pathetically stuck on the human heart, and we have heaped it with a full load of symbolic meaning. A glossary would take up many pages, but we only need to think of a few everyday metaphors to take the point. The heart, as everybody knows, is quintessentially an organ expressing human love. It also carries out a number of specialized subfunctions under this heading, doing duty when required for romantic dalliance, sexual passion, the person of the loved one, or simply as a point of focus for love. But the heart is more than a versatile romantic tool like a Swiss army knife. It can be used to refer to any non-romantic preference, if this is strengthened by emotion ('I set my heart on it . . .'). The heart may also exemplify courage, commitment, zest and essential personality. This perhaps comes from the sense that it is physically *central*, at our core. (*Cor* is the Latin word for heart, but etymologists say this is a coincidence.) Finally, we use the heart as a symbol of the hidden and most deeply personal part of ourselves: a place of inner meditation, our 'heart of hearts'.

So, as a result of the way it is used *symbolically*, the heart is more than a vital life-supporting organ; it is seen as central to our most emotionally-loaded social relationships. The reason why this big muscle has been so important culturally and medically is easy to see. Unlike the other internal organs, the heart is constantly available to us. The stomach, kidneys, bladder and lungs let us know of any discomfort, but otherwise remain largely silent. The heart alone can be continually referred to, eavesdropped upon, interrogated. Moreover, its varying beat reflects our state of exertion, fear and emotion, which is transmitted around the body to wherever the pulse can be felt. It is a portable health-monitor, always hooked up and switched on, and checkable minute by minute. The following lines by Richard Mockton Milnes might be justifiably mistaken for the anthem of a Victorian hypochondriac:

> I wandered by the brookside,
>   I wandered by the mill,
> I could not hear the brook flow,
>   The noisy wheel was still;
> There was no burr of grasshopper
>   No chirp of any bird;
> But the beating of my own heart
>   Was all the sound I heard.

The significance of the *sound* of the heartbeat ('lub-dub' to medical students, but it is expressive enough to be 'tom-tom') cannot be underestimated. As we develop inside the maternal womb, one of our strongest early sensations is the amplified rhythmical thump of the mother's heart. When I hear a recording of the human heartbeat through loudspeakers or (even better) headphones, there is an unmistakable visceral response as my body recognizes the pattern of that first aural contact from another person, my mother. What effect does the rise and fall of the maternal heart have on the foetus? Because a pregnant woman shares her bloodstream with the baby, if she panics, weeps, meditates or makes love, her biochemical reactions will cross into the baby, while simultaneously the heart's rhythm changes. Quickly the foetal nervous system associates blood chemistry changes with rhythmical sound, which means it is conditioned from the earliest possible stage to rhythm which it will later experience as drum-beat, chanting, dancing and music – all powerful evokers of feeling, and great bringers and breakers of calm. Although we have to pay it attention before we become consciously aware of it, our own heartbeat, too, must subliminally exert some slight but constant influence on our emotions – although for the most part the effect is in the other direction.

The mystery of heartbeat evoked imaginative explanation long before it was clear what the heart is actually *doing* as it throbs and slips from side to side in its yellow lubricated envelope. To the ancient Egyptians, for whom physiology was a branch of magic, the heart was simply the symbol of life. When it got tired, life ebbed away. Embalming, the only process by which a person could hope for life after death, involved removal of all the inner organs except for the heart. After death, the heart had to go before Osiris and forty-two judges of the dead, who weighed it in a balance, so that the owner's true character was revealed. To make sure that the departed did themselves justice, a special scarab – the dung-rolling beetle, used so widely in Egyptian art as the symbol of immortal life – would be inscribed with passages from the Book of the Dead. This would be slipped into place under the mummy's bandages just where they covered the heart. The inscriptions were designed to coach the heart in good advocacy, since it was necessary to persuade the gods of its owner's worthiness: 'See, this heart of mine, it weeps in the presence of Osiris and pleads for mercy.' Minus the deity, the line could appear in any modern pop lyric.

The Egyptian tradition also regarded the heart as the location of the emotions and the intellect, as did Aristotle (though not his master, Plato). The Greeks, having inherited and refined the Egyptians' world-picture, gave the heart a prime place in their symbolic system and especially in their poetry, whose interests ranged across the whole spectrum of human emotion. This poetic primacy was transmitted with few alterations down the centuries and is still, imaginatively, part of a living tradition, untouched by science and rationalism.

Before science and reason inherited the earth, the imagination spawned an entire system of medicine based on the centrality of the heart. In due course we shall see echoes of this as modern medicine begins to rediscover this heart/mind complex. But first let us look at a pre-scientific system which has extraordinary power, although in physiological terms it is utterly incorrect.

The humours of the heart

The theory of humours was originally a spin-off from Graeco-Roman physics. This stated that the world is made up of four perfectly balanced *elements* – earth, air, fire and water – which in themselves mix the four essential qualities of cold, heat, moisture and dryness. These elements were thought to correspond to fluids in the body: black bile, blood, yellow bile, and phlegm – the humours. Diseases were considered to arise from imbalances in the humours. The system was perfected by the Roman physician Galen (AD 121–199) whose prestige became so great that he ruled as the presiding genius of medicine for one and a half millennia – until, that is, the time of Galileo and Descartes.

For Galen the body was a four-string fiddle, the humours were the strings and the physician was the one who tried to tune them. All well-being hung on this harmonious adjustment. Each organ was dominated by the different mixtures of qualities, and so by different elements and humours, and our psychological characteristics also were determined by them – hence the adjectives 'melancholic', 'choleric', 'sanguine' and 'phlegmatic'. These terms contained as much meaning for doctors as 'cancer' and 'diabetes' have today.

One final notion must be mentioned, since it came into play when medical men using this system discussed the effect of jangled humours. The Greek Philolaus, a follower of Pythagoras, had long ago explained the phenomenon of life by means of *spirits* which he claimed flowed through the body. These weightless vivifying substances separated living things roughly into three groups, depending on whether one, two or all three of the spirits are present.

The first, *vegetative* or *natural* spirits, were common to all living things, from cabbages to kings. The second, known as *vital* spirits, gave movement and vitality and were possessed by insects, fish, reptiles, birds, beasts and human beings. Thirdly came the *animal* spirits which, despite the name, were possessed only by people, being for the *anima* or soul. In man, according to Galen, natural spirits were manufactured by the liver, which also made blood from food. The blood washed tidally round the body (rather than in Harveian circles) and as it did so it passed the spirits around the body, via the veins, to keep the tissue continually fed. When introduced into the 'furnace' of the heart, however, these vein-carried spirits were charged with extra zest as a result of being mixed with air from the lungs (imagined as bellows). The vital spirits which resulted were then squirted into the arteries and, when they approached the brain, became topped up with the even higher-grade animal spirits, productive of reason and consciousness. These achieved their distribution through the nerve fibres, assumed by Galen to be hollow. The pathological effect of unbalanced humours, then, was to corrupt these indispensable spirits or cause them to leak away.

Historians of science have usually been very hard on the tradition which Galen consummated, seeing it as a crippling influence on the development of 'real' science.[2] Certainly Galen's physiology was factually wide of the mark. He did not realize, for instance, that the heart was a pump, preferring to see it as a furnace which heated and refined the vital spirits. Yet many of his ideas had considerable descriptive power and intellectual appeal, and he was undoubtedly a remarkable anatomist. On the clinical side Galen's system – in theory at any rate – encouraged the doctor to pay very close attention to the whole patient, though in practice his followers were often more inclined to take a few superficial measurements before prescribing with a golden quotation from the Master's writings. But neither Galen nor his system should be held responsible for the laxity of those who came after him.

The conscientious Galenic doctor knew how to take a patient's history, and to relate aspects of personality and psychology to physical symptoms. If faced, for example, with tiredness, angina and shortage of breath he would (quite correctly) look for the cause in the patient's heart. But his first interest would be not the physical state of the heart, which he had no means of looking at, but the patient's state of mind. An illustration is given by Galen himself.

THE CASE OF THE ROMAN GIRL

She was suffering from insomnia, listlessness and fatigue. Her doctors could find nothing the matter and her worried family called in Galen. At the time, a particular dance-troupe (the Roman equivalent of a rock band) was particularly fashionable. Galen noticed during his house-call that, when this group was mentioned in idle conversation, the patient's colour changed. He immediately checked her pulse-rate and found it was raised. He decided to carry out a discreet clinical trial:

> On the next day I said to one of my followers that, when I paid my visit to the woman, he was to come a little later and announce

17

to me, 'Morphus is dancing today'. When he said this I found the pulse was unaffected. Similarly on the next day, when I had an announcement made about another member of the troupe . . . On the fourth evening I kept very careful watch when it was announced that Pylades was dancing and noticed that the pulse was very much disturbed. Thus I found out that the woman was in love with Pylades.

Speculating about how the other doctors had been bamboozled, he could only suppose that 'they have no clear conception of how the body tends to be affected by mental conditions. Possibly they do not know that a pulse is altered by quarrels and alarm which suddenly disturb the mind'.[3]

Judged by Galen's system, the patient's tiredness and depression came not from being in love as such, but from its frustration. The vital spirits are pushed from the blood by a choking excess of black bile in the heart, which also raises the pulse. Under this cold dry influence, the heart gradually begins to wither until, if this continues for a long time, it ceases to function. On autopsy, it will resemble a dried-up pod.

All this is very quaint, very old-world, but what can we learn from a set of fossilized fictions? Well, there is nothing fictitious about Galen's psychology, for one thing. In spite of the fact that psychology has claimed its place as a science, the four humours are still bricked into its foundations. What is aggression if not choler? Depression is entirely consistent with the melancholic humour, and repression with the phlegmatic. Sanguinity – in its extreme form – equates unmistakably with mania. Sanguine and choleric individuals stand in line with all the other extroverts, while melancholics and phlegmatics find themselves in assertiveness training or social skills therapy. The whole style of mind which leads modern psychologists to classify personality types – anal or oedipal, neurotic or psychotic, convergent or divergent, Type A or Type B, even winners and losers – is utterly in the Galenic tradition.

But there is another more powerful reason for Galen's continued relevance, for he was the originator of the *allopathic* approach to medicine.

Allopathy

The word was first used by the inventor of homeopathy Samuel Hahnemann (1755–1843), to refer to the guiding principle behind the orthodox medicine of his day, and to underline the contrast with his own theories. He defined allopathy as 'the curing of a diseased action by the inducing of another or a different action, yet not necessarily diseased'. Allopathy is based on the notion of balance, and on countering imbalance by vigorous and positive expert intervention. This took either of two forms. The doctor might *introduce* substances into the body to counteract the noxious influence of disease – by drugs, feeding, heating or cooling the patient. Or he might *deprive* the body of something, or perhaps shift substances around within it. This could be by means of purging, bloodletting, sweating, amputating, cupping or starving, always with the object of restoring balance. The flaw in this approach is that, once you start throwing treatments on to a balance, the scales may begin to oscillate this way and that, calling for increasingly energetic and grosser counter-measures to maintain control. The result is polypragmacy – the use of not just one but a selection-box of therapies – and, especially, to *polypharmacy*, which entails the use of highly complicated medicinal compounds sometimes containing scores of ingredients.

Roman, Medieval and Renaissance doctors made extraordinary use of multiple drugs. A prescription would contain, at a minimum, an active chemical agent, an ingredient to counteract its side-effects, an adjuvant to back up the active agent, something to counteract the adjuvant's side-effects, a general tonic and perhaps a bowel tonic. But even this would be a modest 'economy' medicament. Louis XIII of France, a hypochondriac on a royal scale, is said to have been bled almost once a week and, in the course of a single year, to have been dosed with over 200 purgatives and the same number of enemas. Since these medicines are likely to have been patent amalgamations of all sorts of chemicals, it is quite impossible to estimate the quantity or strength of those which must have passed through the kingly stomach.

Multiple drugs passed into the collective mind of the Western world, and remain a fixed part of patients' own assessments of their medical needs. Before this century people violently distrusted doctors, though they maintained a passionate belief in the effectiveness of strong drugs. They would dose themselves with a vast range of remedies containing quite dangerous poisons such as mercury and arsenic. In the Victorian and Edwardian era, to produce a 'medicinal compound' and back it up with sufficiently grandiose claims might mean to get rich very quickly indeed, as H. G. Wells described in *Tono-Bungay* and more recently The Scaffold in their version of the old army song about 'Lily the Pink', whose bottled salvation was 'most efficacious in every case'.

During the period beween the wars the self-dosing tradition fell into disrepute. There is today, however, a renewed alienation from official medicine and much resort to 'alternative' remedies – mega-vitamins, evening primrose oil, aromatic oils, zinc, selenium, biochemic salts or whatever. However, as in previous periods, it is always recognized that the really strong medicines are in the gift of the medical profession. So, as the historian of medicine Edward Shorter notes, 'One factor troubling doctor-patient relations in our time is that many patients show up with their own diagnoses and prescriptions. They are merely obliged to go to the doctor so that he can write it out for them'.[4] Although this may, at the moment, be more prevalent in North America, studies in Britain show that two-thirds of patients are disappointed if the consultation does not end with a prescription. The patient's demands for such strong drugs as antibiotics (even for viral infections on which they have no effect) and for psycho-active drugs shows how far we would have to travel before freeing patients from the Galenic allopathic mentality.

But before any doctor too quickly tut-tuts over these misguided patients, it must be remembered that polypharmacy is widely practised by doctors themselves, even without the influence of patient demand. To illustrate this, I return to the main subject of this chapter, heart disease. What follows is a paraphrase of a case reported in *The Lancet*. The patient was treated in Glasgow between 1979 and 1986, and I shall call her Mrs Ross.

She is sixty-five years old and was admitted to hospital with congestive heart failure, having had a long history of heart disease. The mitral valve controlling the flow of oxygenated blood from the lungs, through the left-side atrium (auricle or upper chamber) and into the left-side ventricle (lower chamber) had stiffened and narrowed. This causes congestion in the heart and greatly increases blood pressure in the pulmonary artery, where the slowed-down blood backs up like a traffic jam into the lungs. The result is breathlessness and sometimes the coughing of blood.

In 1979 Mrs Ross had cardiac surgery to fit her with an artificial mitral valve. But this was ineffective and she needed several more admissions to hospital in the next few years. By November 1984 she was suffering from abdominal oedema (also called ascites) – a result of her damaged circulation – and was taking diuretics to counter this: initially frusemide and later spironolactone. In addition she was on digoxin, derived from the heart drug digitalis, and the subject of a recent *Lancet* editorial which suggested that, though invaluable in the acute phase of heart illness, digoxin is ineffective in the medium-to-long term. In addition, according to one patient – a scientist involved in space research writing to *The Lancet* – long-term digoxin in his case resulted in 'several after-effects, the most important being a dulling of the mental process' which, until he was taken off it after a year, caused him to consider taking early retirement through mental disablement.[7] Apart from the diuretics and digoxin, Mrs Ross's medication included daily thyroxine (thyroid hormone), warfarin (anti-coagulant), and mianserin (anti-depressant).

Now her doctors added captopril, a strong last-resort drug designed to lower blood pressure. The captopril successfully brought the blood pressure down, but Mrs Ross was still not feeling too well and the oedema did not disperse. However, the pharmacy had not yet shot its bolt. Her drug intake was augmented with an even stronger diuretic, metolazone, and this did reduce the excess abdominal fluid as Mrs Ross lost seven pounds in weight. But now she complained of nausea with loss of appetite, and of generally feeling very ill. This was because her kidneys – already weakened by her medical condition, had failed as a result of the metolazone interacting with the captopril. Both the latter drugs were discontinued, relieving the kidneys. But poor Mrs Ross still had her congested heart condition, high blood pressure, oedema, breathlessness and, perhaps, the mental confusion that can go with digoxin.

As a layman, I cannot be alone in thinking Mrs Ross's case a medical horror story. Yet to insiders of hospital medicine it would hardly raise an eyebrow. It is, quite simply, an everyday routine affair.

If Mrs Ross's case illustrates how modern allopathy typically struggles with heart disease, it clearly shows which parts of the Galenic tradition have been preserved. These are the parts which emphasized piecemeal intervention against symptoms, the use of specific medicines to deal with these, the use of further measures to counteract the ill-effects of the specifics and in general a reliance on tackling each difficulty, each new symptom or side-effect, as it arises. This kind of acute medicine is a juggling act. Other aspects of Galen – the 'holistic' approach, the importance of an overall assessment, the contact with the patient over a period of time – were discarded in the hey-day of mechanistic medicine, although there are clear signs that some individuals in the medical professions are now looking for their revival.

The causes of heart disease

Mrs Ross's mitral valve may very well have been damaged by rheumatic heart disease. This would result from an infection several years earlier which injured the heart's valvular tissue, and prepared the way for a later failure. However, this is not the cause of the epidemic of heart disease which has afflicted humanity – in particular, northern humanity – in this century.

Epidemic is not an inaccurate word. In 1983, the rate of hospital admissions for heart disease in England per 100,000 of the population was well over double what it had been twenty-five years earlier. By comparison, hospital admissions for cerebrovascular disease (strokes) were up by only 40 per cent. Of the 102,130 men under sixty-five who died in 1984, one quarter succumbed to ischaemic heart disease which, when you consider all the possible causes of death from accident to the various cancers, is a menacing proportion. But some of the details can be puzzling. Incidence of the disease in women has also increased, though as a cause of premature death it is at less than half the male level. Women seem to be relatively protected from heart disease by the female hormone oestrogen, and it is only after the menopause that their incidence of the disease begins to catch up with that of men. But this hormonal protection is only part of the story.

Ischaemic heart disease is the condition we normally associate with the phrase *heart attack*, i.e. a sudden failure of the energy-carrying blood supply to the heart muscle, though often it is a chronic rather than an acute condition. These days the most fashionable explanation for the disease is that high levels of cholesterol in the bloodstream cause a gradual narrowing of the coronary arteries, leaving them vulnerable to blockage by a blood clot. Such a blockage cuts off the supply of oxygenated blood to the heart muscle: a serious but variable condition, depending on the part of the muscle affected. It may result in total stoppage of the heart, or it may cause disturbances to the heart's rhythm, with breathlessness and pain. There is no pain arising in the heart itself, which like many internal organs has no pain receptors. 'Heart ache' cannot physiologically exist. Instead the pain is referred (i.e. transferred) to nerves in the chest, giving the characteristic pain of angina which is regularly mistaken for severe indigestion.

Mapping the epidemic

So who runs the greatest risk of heart disease? The people who can best tell us are not the hospital doctors and family practitioners. They see heart patients, no two the same, day in day out. But they are too rushed, too absorbed in 'firefighting' the symptoms to look systematically for the common underlying truths. So we turn to the medical map-makers, the epidemiologists. These certainly do have answers, though they are not framed from studies of individual cases of the disease, or by biochemical work on the blood or the heart cells. They are purely statistical averages – culled from hundreds of thousands of questionnaires designed to help compare the lives and habits of heart patients with those of people with healthy hearts.

23

Thus the epidemiologist defines not a *cause*, but a number of statistically significant *risk factors*. In the absence of an adequate explanation, these risk factors must do duty as signposts.

Statistically then, those most at risk are, in no particular order: males, smokers, the obese and those with high blood pressure. So far, so easy. All these can be identified and warned. But there are others, less easy to spot: those with high levels of cholesterol in the blood stream, those eating high-fat diets, people living in developed Western economies, *poor* people living in those economies, people who sit down a lot, people under particular types of stress, members of previously cohesive but now splintered social groups, people with particular character traits. Now we are getting into murkier water. No one is saying that any of these things necessarily *cause* heart disease, they are simply associated with it statistically. How can we sort out the variables?

For instance, if a heart attack hits a man who has been driven by a personality trait and/or by the stress of his (sedentary) job to smoke sixty cigarettes a day, who can tell whether the personality, the stress, the smoking or the lack of exercise is the cause of his disease? If they all contributed (*multifactorial* causation, which is the buzz-word today), in what proportion did they do so? Which should he give up first, the smoking or the long hours on the telephone? Which should be adopted first, the low-fat diet or jogging?

The Royal College of Physicians, reporting on 250 deaths under the age of 50 years in 1979, noted that 98 were cases of self-destruction. These included 8 suicides, 6 alcoholics with cirrhosis of the liver, 13 heavy smokers with lung cancer and, 'Among those whose death was attributable to myocardial infarction (31) there were 25 with one or more causal factors within their own control. Twelve were grossly overweight; 22 smoked large numbers of cigarettes; 2 diabetics and 2 hypertensives did not comply with their treatment; and 3 others had had symptoms for a long time before they consulted a doctor'.

The authors added, rather primly, that, 'Doctors have been saying for years that the causes of many of the killing diseases of middle life are not mysteries, but are contributed to by overeating, excess alcohol and tobacco.' They then note that members of Social Class One have cut their heart attack risk by more than half since before the war, while the number of heart attacks in the population as a whole has more than doubled. Their conclusion is 'that people in Social Class One do heed such advice, whereas other groups do not'.[8]

If this is true, some kind of decision to *refuse* heart disease must have been taken by the wealthiest class – an effort of mind made to *stop killing themselves*, with cumulative effects on the statistics collected over the next forty years. Equally, no such decision can have been taken by the working class.

There are numerous questions going begging in all this, but the class issue and the self-destruction issue must detain us. The Black Report of 1980 into *Inequalities in Health* in Britain shows the factual truth behind the Royal College's assumptions: the poorer you are, the worse your health. Sir Douglas Black, however, did not endorse the College's quasi-Victorianisms about the feckless self-destructiveness of the lower orders. For him, the blame was a complex mixture of occupational differences, economic pressures, educational inequality and 'deprivation in its various forms'.

A well-known study of workers in the British Civil Service[9] indicates the place of class among the risk factors for heart disease. Between 1969 and 1976, Whitehall Civil Servants of all grades who died before retirement were counted and, when the figures were analysed, the most striking variations were discovered between the death-rates in the different grades. Some would suppose, knowing the association between rich diets, stress and heart attacks, that 'top' people would get more of them. In fact, for every one who died from a heart attack in the highest grade, four died in the lowest grade. Assuming that the well-known behavioural risk factors (diet, smoking, lack of exercise, hypertension) could account for the difference, the researchers were surprised to find that, when these were taken into account, *three out of five* heart attacks were still unexplained and indeed could not have been predicted on any known scale of risk.

The whole risk factor story is beset with such difficulties. So, although knowledge of the risks clearly creates useful reference points, healers have to make their own, more personal, maps of the patients' lives. Heart disease, like the game of cricket, cannot be understood by staring at the averages. Disease is a personal event, determined by complex and subtle psychological factors which constantly elude the calculator and the computer program.

Hurry and worry

There is one set of general findings which throws strong light on the psychology of heart disease. It has been realized by physiologists for most of this century that mental *stress* causes biochemical changes in the body. This is a system designed to save our lives. For instance, on any normal morning I awake in a sleep-sodden trance, dragging myself unwillingly towards consciousness and that first cup of tea. But if I were to open my bleary eye to the sight of flames dancing up the curtains, I would be out of my bed in a jackknife's flash, fully alert and fully functioning. Walter Cannon, in his influential *The Wisdom of the Body*, described these 'fight and flight' mechanisms in 1914. Immediately it distinguishes a threat, the mind triggers adrenalin- and cortisol-release from the adrenal glands, which sit on top of the kidneys. We can feel this as 'butterflies', but its covert effects are much more radical – a complete and sudden change in the body's chemistry and the activation of our emergency services. Glycogen is released from the liver, which boosts the blood's sugar (and energy) content; the pupils of the eyes dilate, improving vision in the dark; the heart rate and blood pressure increase, forcing more oxygenated blood into the brain and enhancing its performance; blood drains from the gut and is diverted into the limb muscles; non-essential services such as digestion are closed down; hair muscles and sweat glands start to work; and, finally, the blood's efficiency in forming clots becomes sharper.

This is – or should be – a sleeping volcano in the body, erupting rarely and only when strictly necessary. But, being a mind-activated mountain, the volcano can be triggered by thought alone and this happens often and inappropriately in many people. Chronic hostility and a sense of being under threat, which may be experienced over a long period, causes a continuous flow of glucocorticoids, strong substances which particularly affect protein, fat and carbohydrate metabolism. What effect does this have on the body?

First, and obviously, excitement can be *exciting*. But through conditioning it may also become addictive. The compulsive gambler is a victim to this addiction, longing for the next squirt of self-administered adrenalin main-lined into his bloodstream. Probably sky-divers, mountaineers, hang-gliders, racing drivers, fox-hunters – even actors and politicians – are prey to the same craving. But to some extent, we all enjoy stress.

Second, chronic stress brings adaptive responses into play. The body initiates long-term changes designed to cope with new, higher levels of biochemical excitation. But according to the theory of Hans Selye, the Canadian 'father' of stress research, this adaptation cannot be sustained indefinitely. If stress is continued, and especially if it increases, a breakdown is inevitable. In laboratory animals this leads to precipitate death.

The relevance of this to people and their heart attacks interested Californian cardiologists Meyer Friedman and Ray Rosenman in the late sixties. As soon as they started to look for it, they saw that the phenomenon had been blindingly obvious. The pace of consultation at their clinic was being dictated – was being *hurried* – not, as would be usual, by the punishing clinical schedule of two busy physicians, but by the *patients*. The seats in the waiting room were worn only at the front edge. Why? Because the patients' physical posture, as they waited, betrayed their internal states. They were *on edge*, always eager to be away, anxious to waste no time, with many unmissable appointments, calls to make, memos to dictate. How could such people sit back and relax as they waited their turn?

Friedman and Rosenman called them the Type A people, as opposed to the rest of the population, who were Type B. Type As are always on hot bricks, or else under the gun: time-urgent, impatient, competitive. They are driven by ambition, thwarted or otherwise, and a sense of threat which they meet with feelings of strong hostility. This does not mean they must be toweringly dominant individuals. The White Rabbit in *Alice in Wonderland* is a perfect Type A rabbit and yet, as Lewis Carroll wrote in an article on 'Alice on the Stage': 'I am sure his voice should quaver, and his knees quiver, and his whole air suggest a total inability to say "Bo!" to a goose'.[10]

Initially, Friedman and Rosenman performed some extremely successful laboratory experiments to test their hypothesis that the White Rabbit is more prone to heart disease than, for example, the Dormouse. Recent research into a real-life situation has supported the idea that Type As have different cardiovascular stress responses Type Bs. In a study of students facing final exams carried out recently at Lancashire Polytechnic, Type As had a consistently higher rise in blood pressure and heart rate than Type Bs.

This study was intended to analyse and clarify a number of things about Types A and B, including heart rate, blood pressure, feelings and coping strategies. For instance, as the exams approached, the students' minor ailments gave rise to many more doctor visits for Type Bs than Type As, though the reported levels of illness were the same. The latter were more likely to retain control in their own hands, by treating themselves. This internalized, active approach to coping by Type As was also in evidence in other ways. As the stress increased, the Type As smoked significantly more (though no students initially selected for the trial had been heavy smokers), while the Bs were more likely to resort to alcohol to relieve the pressure. Again this is interpreted by the psychologists as a difference between preparing for a threat actively (nicotine used as a stimulant) as compared with the passive approach of dulling the perceived threat with alcohol.[11]

In spite of the promising early work on Type A personality and heart disease, recent research into the link has proved more ambiguous. If, as Rosenman and Friedman originally believed, there is a connection between Type A behaviour and the artery disease which so often precedes heart attacks, it has not yet been convincingly demonstrated. As a result the Type A mentality has itself come under analysis, to see if any of its *parts* can be isolated as the main heart attack risk. Now, one of these elements in the Type A profile, *hostility*, has begun to be regarded as the crucial factor. The Lancashire study showed hostility to be very significantly different between the two types, as compared, for example, with anxiety. But when anger was studied at Duke University in Carolina, an interesting sub-variation was discovered among Type As themselves. To quote the researchers, the 'level of hostility was unrelated to coronary heart disease in those patients who disclosed a willingness to express anger or hostility openly against the source of frustration'.[12]

28

The original conception of Type A behaviour, then, has had to be refined. Ambition, competitiveness or anxiety about time may not in themselves be so dangerous to the heart, unless accompanied (as they so often are) by anger, distrust and resentment. Coping may also be particularly important. As far as heart attack risk is concerned, Type A people are now being subdivided into those who express themselves well, and who are said to be less at risk, and those who fail to express themselves and so attract more risk. The fussy crossness of the White Rabbit clearly suggests he was of the latter.

Certainly, a constant 'on guard' mentality results in higher levels of adrenalin in the blood, which is known to assist blood clotting. Other circulating hormones released or triggered by the grumbling volcano of anger may help to cause the arterial narrowing, perhaps through some change in the fatty content of the blood.

The broken heart

Quite apart from the choleric heart, there is also the shock of bereavement or other loss. Looked at culturally, this is particularly loathsome to the heart. It is *taken* to heart, and it *breaks* the heart.

The small Italian community of Roseto, Pennsylvania, was studied by heart disease epidemiologists in 1962. Despite their high-fat diets (and many fat bodies) they had a much lower heart disease rate than neighbouring towns. The suggestion was that their settled tight-knit community, imported intact from the Mediterranean, helped to insulate them from the epidemic of coronary heart disease then at its height in the United States. If this were true, those who moved away – it was reasoned – should lose their advantage. And this is exactly the finding of the research workers. Rosetans who went to work elsewhere were found to have heart disease risks closer to the national average.[13]

In the same way settlers in America from Japan (where there is a very low rate of heart disease) find their coronary risk rising to the American average. In Britain there are even more interesting findings like this. It has only recently come to light that the mortality from heart disease among Asians is much higher than in the general population. This is in spite of Asians smoking less and eating a much 'healthier' diet, low in saturated fats and high in fibre and polyunsaturates. Indian migrants to Fiji, South Africa, Singapore and Trinidad also have a higher than expected rate of heart attacks.[14]

It is interesting to note that the United States, which has borne the brunt of this century's heart disease epidemic (proportionately 27 per cent worse at its height in the sixties than the worst British figures from the seventies) has also been the greatest social melting-pot of all time. Now that heart disease is falling sharply there, we might at least speculate that this is something to do with the dying off of the last generation of immigrants. The disruptions of migration, the encounter with racism and a new kind of poverty, and the social amputation from the mother culture . . . perhaps these are capable of causing some kind of hidden grief reaction, the ill-effects of which fall on the heart.

Such perspectives on heart disease make it impossible to see the heart simply as the kind of mechanical component described at the beginning of this chapter and I hope I have shown that such perspectives are justified by what doctors are learning about the circumstances of heart disease. Even the idea of 'a broken heart' seems more literal than metaphorical again. The observation that recently bereaved men have something like twice the 'normal' rate of heart attacks gives some statistical support to the idea. The feeling of bereavement was described by C. S. Lewis, writing about the death of his wife:

No one ever told me that grief felt so like fear. I am not afraid, but the sensation is like being afraid. The same fluttering in the stomach, the same restlessness, the yawning. I keep on swallowing.[15]

Lewis's grief is palpably a mental agony, yet it is also, as these words testify, physiological and hormonal. Later we shall consider hormones in greater detail. But the notion of a relationship between the hormones and the personality – and especially the emotions – is fully justified by what we know about the brain's regulation of the body's chemistry. This link between the emotions and the constituents of the blood (the latter being a major factor in the cause of heart disease) provide a possible reason why the heart is so susceptible to the emotions and why heart disease is linked to them.

Galen would have been delighted with this information. Experiences which *moved* humours around the heart (causing 'emotion') were for him the main instigators of disease; love, anger and grief were regarded medically as particularly dangerous for the heart. So in modern accounts of the relationship between the emotions and heart disease we are not so very far, after all, from the theory of humours, whereby an excess of choler burst the heart and too much melancholy choked it.

The heart is of primal importance to our lives, both objectively and subjectively. The effect of modern medicine has been to keep these two aspects strictly separated and to deal only with the objective. Yet the bankruptcy of the reductionist approach to heart disease is increasingly apparent: until the subjectivity associated with the heart is allowed to recombine in harmony with our objective knowledge, the prospect of understanding heart disease remains remote.

Chapter 2

Pain

**'That which makes us endure pain with such
impatience is that we are not accustomed to
take our chief contentment in the soul'**
Montaigne

---

*T*he heart is superficially one of the most objective entities in
the human body; pain is among the most subjective. If I survey
pain as I would a territory, perhaps from aerial photographs, I
see a region whose features are all extreme – not a plain, nor
even a vale of tears, but something more like a chain of Gothic
mountains, dark and spiked, with sharp peaks and deep gulfed
valleys, the whole only partly visible through a pall of low
obscuring cloud.

Pain is among the most usual motives for calling in or calling
on a general practitioner. But like depression, another of the
most common complaints heard in surgeries, it is insistent and
intractably *private*. So what a patient says about the pain is the
only way in which a doctor can know it.

Doctors employ a variety of strategems to get round this
problem. Words they treat with suspicion, as not particularly
reliable signposts to pain. On the other hand, posture and facial
expression are excellent indicators of a person's state of mind,
therefore observation of these often tells more. Further details
yet may be extracted from the play of gestures. The way in
which a hand indicates pain – by prodding towards the spot
with an index finger, or knocking at it with a tightly clenched
first – can be more revealing than to say, 'it hurts under my ribs'.
The characteristic pain from a kidney stone radiates spirally
downwards 'from loin to groin' and, as Jonathan Miller tells
us[1], while trying to describe this movement in words patients
sometimes position a hand on the side, with the thumb at the

back and the fingers pointing downwards in front. So, as Miller says, 'the skilled physician can learn a lot from the pantomime of complaint.' Perhaps somebody should write a dictionary of medical body language.

However, neither seeing the pantomime nor hearing the verbal description can really be described as sharing the patient's experience, for in reality pain can never be truly shared. My pain is a restricted area: the only one with a pass is me. This makes it extremely barren soil for the cultivation of scientific explanations. Tumours and toenails can be inspected, counted, measured and modelled. Tummy bugs and tennis elbow can be assessed against the performance norms of the bowel or the overhead smash. Pain has no such reference points, it can only be approached by proxy.

So, since its experience can neither be meaningfully shared nor usefully compared, the physician is forced to take it as read, prescribe some palliative treatment, before looking for whatever intervention will remove the cause of pain: abolition of an infection, support of a sprain, the correction of a habit of life.

This is fine where doctors do not automatically react to the presentation of pain as if it were nothing but a language of clues, cryptic or otherwise, to encode information about organic disease. Such a reaction may satisfy many patients: but what if the runes cannot be deciphered?

Descartes's burglar alarm

Pain has always mounted a dual challenge to the intellect. Firstly, there is the doctor's question: 'How can we match the experience of pain to the reality of disease?' And secondly, there is the moral philosopher's problem: 'How can the world be good if it contains pain?' Much of the power of a seventeenth-century 'mechanistic' philosophy like that of René Descartes came from its ability to dissolve the difference between these problems in an overall model of reality, whose justification was its 'perfectly balanced' design. To him, the universe was an automaton, a majestic piece of clockwork wound up and left to tick by God. Pain, to Descartes, was simply a part of the mechanism. He was not over-interested in its morality or immorality. He argued that, if the creator lumbered us with

33

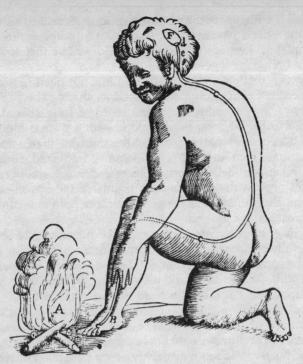

Fig. 1. Descartes' (1664) concept of the pain pathway.

pain, fair's fair, he amply compensated by giving us pleasure. But Descartes' idea actually devalued pain and pleasure both ethically and emotionally. They became no more than quantities heaped on each side of the divinity's scrupulous scales.

The difference between Descartes' and Galen's idea of balance is instructive. Descartes' balance is that of a flywheel; if out of balance, it works inefficiently or not at all. Only the *quantity* of its output is affected. Galen's balance is more that of music, where the *quality* is all. Changes in balance (harmony) are possible without destroying the whole, and may even enhance it. Only gross, sustained and willed imbalance is destructive. Thus there is a place for freedom, a place for the mind in the Galenic tradition which Descartes' system could not admit. There mind was banished, along with soul, into a separate and insulated room.

So in the Cartesian body-machine (a working component in

his universe-machine) pain had a simple function: to warn of danger, damage or disequilibrium in some part of the machine. Such simplicity of purpose is matched by an equally facile mechanism.

'When I feel pain in my foot,' says Descartes in his *Sixth Meditation*, 'physics tells me that the feeling is passed on by the nerves distributed in the foot, which, being stretched like strings from there to the brain, when they are pulled in the foot, simultaneously pull the same place in the brain where they originate and end'.[2] This sketch of pain's action employs the laws of force and motion as if the nerve fibres were a bell-pull, tugged by experience and pealing a chime in the brain.

Descartes' model is seductive, being easy to grasp and until quite recently fitting the conventional objective wisdom well enough to be serviceable. It supposes that all pain is an automatic mechanism, like – to bring the analogy into this century – a burglar alarm. Some unwelcome stimulus, for example a burglar's foot, activates the system's pressure pads, which are distributed throughout the house and linked by wires to an alarm box. The bell rings and the system, registering damage or danger at the site of the pressure pad, takes the appropriate action, such as routing an automatic call through to the police station. On this analogy, the pressure pads are *dedicated pain receptors* located in the body tissue. The connecting wires are the nerve fibres and the alarm box is some *specific pain centre* in the brain. This view has undergone refinement, but even in the 1970s as the 'specificity theory' of pain, it was being taught in medical schools. The trouble is, it does not fit the facts.

Nerves and nerve action

In classical Western medicine there are two great communication networks in the body. Firstly, a canal-system of blood vessels transports chemicals between the cells and organs where they are required either to do certain work or to be worked upon by other chemicals. Secondly, a telephone grid of nerve cells carries news up to and around the brain, and brings away from it the brain's interpretations and instructions. Galen thought that the nervous system, which had been recognised as such in ancient times, was in fact another canal system, carrying the 'animal spirits'. More accurate knowledge of the nerves became possible when, in 1786, Luigi Galvani discovered that an electric charge could make a frog's muscles jump. This cleared the block in understanding and gradually it was understood that electricity flows through the nerve network. An analogy that was not yet available, but would seem appropriate, is that of the telephone wire.

However, further discoveries in the late nineteenth century (just as Alexander Graham Bell was inventing the telephone) show how misleading this analogy is. True, the immensely complicated forking-pathway structure of the nervous system is a relay system of strands along which currents run. But it is not at all like a telephone grid. The current in a telephone wire is continually changing to match the modulating sound waves as they strike the diaphragm in the mouthpiece. There is no uninterrupted modulation of impulse in the nervous system.

The nerve cell, or neuron, is a tree-shaped structure (with roots, trunk and branches) at whose base is the cell body. This, complete with a nucleus, drives the cell's activity. The nucleus is fed by a system of roots, called dendrites, which are distributed throughout the surrounding matter, and these roots pick up news of a stimulus – a flash of light to an optic nerve, a pinprick to one of the skin's receptors – and conveys it to the nucleus. But the cell will only react if the stimulus is strong enough to cross the cell's reaction threshold and, if it does so, the cell is said to 'fire'. Then an impulse is released up the treetrunk – called an axon – and along the branches until, inevitably, it encounters a *synapse* – a junction point with a dendrite feeding the next neuron in the chain.

The synapse consists of a tiny gap between the end of the axon and the next cell's receptor, and this gap – a millionth of an inch across – must be traversed if the impulse is to continue on its journey. It is tempting to think of this as the electrical spark itself, flashing across from terminal to terminal like some microscopic Frankenstein apparatus. But in fact, the electrical signal stops at the frontier – the synapse – and its energy pushes a chemical out like a ferryboat across the gap from cell to cell. It is this chemical – the neurotransmitter – which on arrival affects the nucleus of the next neuron. The impulse continues on its way, each nerve cell acting like a domino in a 'domino-run': as it fires, the domino falls, passing the impulse on to the next cell.

In this way, along many nerve cells bundled together as thick, visible 'afferent' fibres, the painful news travels from the place where the original receptors picked it up to the main trunk route along the spinal cord. From here, it may either continue on up to the brain or bounce automatically back along a 'reflex arc' to an appropriate muscle, where a reflex action (not part of any conscious mental process) will occur in the form of a bodily jerk, a covering motion by the hand or a blink.

So far, nothing contradicts the specificity (burglar-alarm) theory, but as soon as we look and think more carefully two main objections surface. For one thing, there is no pain centre: virtually, it seems, the *whole brain* is involved in processing pain, including its centres for movement-control, the release of glandular secretions, instinct, emotion, body-image, memory and reasoning. As we shall see later, the brain cannot be mapped into a pattern of interlocking departments like a bureaucracy, each charged with the administration of a single discrete function. But even if it could, pain would be an inter-departmental matter disseminated along numerous quite different pathways, informing and informed *by* the whole system.

The second objection to the burglar-alarm theory is that often the subjective experience of pain is not like this at all.

Pains that are not 'there'

A doctor-patient was seen by the eminent neurologist W. K. Livingston in 1926, suffering from paralysis and pain in hand and arm:[3]

Sometimes he had a boring sensation in the bones of the index finger. The sensation seemed to start at the tip of the finger and ascend to the extremity of the shoulder . . . He was frequently nauseated when the pain was at its height. As the pain gradually faded, the sense of tenseness in the hand eased somewhat, but never in a sufficient degree to permit it to be moved. In the intervals beween the sharper attacks of pain, he experienced a persistent burning in the hand. The sensation was not unbearable and at times he could be diverted so as to forget it for short intervals. When it became annoying a hot towel thrown over his shoulder or a drink of whisky gave him partial relief.

A conventional first approach to such a problem might be to make a close visual and manual examination of the hand and arm, take X-rays and put the hand through a series of checks on the circulation and suchlike. Livingston did none of these – for the simple reason that his patient's 'hand' no longer existed. Nor did his arm; it had been amputated just below the shoulder several years earlier.

Yet for the unfortunate patient, the hand, the arm, their posture and the pains he felt in them were exactly as if the limb were still attached to his body. Questioning him, Livingston was curious about the strong emphasis he placed on the tension he perceived in his phantom. The patient offered to demonstrate his discomfort to Livingston:

> He asked me to clench my fingers over my thumb, flex my wrist and raise the arm into a hammerlock position and hold it there. He kept me in this position as long as I could stand it. At the end of five minutes I was perspiring freely, my hand and arm felt unbearably cramped and I quit. *But you can take your hand down*, he said.

Horatio Nelson believed that his continued consciousness of the arm shot away by French chain-shot was proof of the existence of the soul. Be that as it may, the mind has a sharp feeling of bodily existence, including an awareness of the position of the limbs which is quite independent of the eyes, ears and sense of touch. It is as if the physical body throws a shadow over the mind, giving a template for the body-image.

Now it is well-known that amputees like Nelson are usually aware of their missing limb, just as if it had not been removed. The arm is felt to tingle, move and swing with the body's movement and can even be consciously stretched out to grasp something. Why the ghost of a missing limb should continue to linger so disturbingly is not properly understood. It is generally regarded as a purely mental phenomenon, an after-image which very gradually fades and changes, losing definite shape, over the remains of a lifetime. The existence of unbearable pain in the phantom limb, however, is even more bizarre, 'a thing wondrous strange and prodigious' as one early medical writer,

Ambroise Pare, said in 1552. Nelson was not afflicted with that, but he was in a fortunate minority. Most amputees suffer some form of phantom pain.

The case of Joseph Corless

Equally hard to deal with is the horrible condition of *causalgia*. This is often the sequel to traumatic nerve damage from a bullet wound and is felt as not just a burning but a 'blazing' pain which usually continues for more than six months. The case of Joseph Corless, an American Civil War soldier shot in the left arm, illustrates the horror of such pain syndromes. Corless's pain, accompanied by extreme skin sensitivity all along the forearm and in the hand, started two days after the injury. Two years later it was still undiminished. S. W. Mitchell described the patient's pathetic attempts to minimize irritation to his hand and arm, an account which in itself is agonizing:

> He keeps his hand wrapped in a rag, wetted with cold water, and covered with oiled silk, and even tucks the rag carefully under the flexed fingers tips . . . He will allow no one to touch his skin, save with a wetted hand, and even then he is careful to exact careful manipulation. He keeps a bottle of water about him and carries a sponge in his right hand. This hand he wets before he handles anything; used dry it hurts the other limb . . . He thus describes the pain at its height: *It is as if a rough bar of iron were thrust to and fro through the knuckles, a red-hot iron placed at the junction of the palm and thumb, with a heavy weight on it, and the skin being rasped off my finger ends.*

Phantom limb pain and causalgia do not spring directly from the original limb injuries, though of course injury or disease are the remote causes. Unlike most pain experiences, they result not from painful sensory inputs but the *loss* of input following damage to the nerve. Absent or mangled, the nerve cannot contribute to the normal balance of sensory activity in the central nervous system. Thus the system as a whole finds itself incomplete, and by way of protest it manufactures severe pain at the place where the missing sensory activity should be originating. Paraplegics also experience appalling pain from parts of their body where there is no normal sensory input, and for the same reason. Pain is now not a cry of alarm but a shriek of loss, almost of grief, from the organism as a whole for its missing part. It follows that treatment which tries to isolate the painful area – for example by cutting nerves – may often worsen the imbalance of sensory input and paradoxically increase the pain.

There are other kinds of loss, and pain is their mode of expression; not as common as tears, but as telling. In our everyday language we freely allow the idea of emotional pain, but we usually think of this usage as largely a metaphor which takes the idea of 'real' bodily pain to represent mental or spiritual suffering. Perhaps by and large it is so. But consider Mr K.

The case of Mr K.

This man, aged thirty-six, had had left-sided facial pain for one year. *Tic doloureux* was excluded and he was sent to a psychotherapist, Dr Allan Walters, with a referral for 'atypical facial neuralgia, likely psychogenic'. Walters' method[4] was to look for a psychological trigger, and he found one by using association tests: the man's pain was evoked by symbols of being alone, especially by an empty seat beside him in the cinema.

It transpired that, until twelve months earlier, Mr K. had been in the habit of drinking so heavily that his first wife had left him. He had remarried, but his drunkenness continued until one night he quarrelled with his second wife. In a fury, she threw herself at him, threatened to leave and at the same time swung at and slapped his left cheek. He then stopped drinking and the pains began.

Dr Walters reports that 'the pain vanished temporarily with sodium amytal, one grain, intravenously, and he recovered completely with psychotherapy and rehabilitation. His wife was co-operative and he was assisted with his alcoholism.'

Freud would have called Mr K.'s pain 'conversion hysteria', by which he would have meant that the unbearable thought of loss was suppressed and unconsciously converted into a self-punitive pain. Whether or not hysteria or neurosis were actually present, Mr K. was using pain at least partially as a form of expression, as he had once used alcohol. But it is a more private language than alcoholism – more private than any form of overtly inappropriate or anti-social behaviour, which is meant to be seen and understood by other people. It is certainly more private than the production of psoriasis or urticaria.

This personal communication with himself was highly complicated, referring to at least three matters which were on Mr K.'s unconscious mind. Remember, he had been alcoholic even before the end of his first marriage. But he had discovered that his two emotional props were mutually exclusive, since it is an axiom that pathological drinking is a solitary activity and usually incompatible with any kind of successful marriage or relationship. His first wife's departure had already told him this. His second wife made it explicit: he must choose between her and the bottle. So his facial neuralgia – which was evoked by the empty cinema seat and associated feelings of aloneness – had three linked messages for him. Firstly, it reminded him of the pain of solitude. Secondly, it continued the slap which had stopped his access to alcohol. And thirdly, it offered a substitute for the alocholism itself.

Allan Walters' considerable experience of psychogenic pain led him to conclude that it is generally to be regarded as a way of expressing – a satisfaction of the *need* to express – some buried and unbearable thought. The great majority of such pain is felt in the head, neck and upper body.

'Pain,' said the nineteenth-century surgeon Leriche, 'is not a simple affair of an impulse travelling at a fixed rate along a nerve. It is the result of a conflict between a stimulus and the whole individual.' Or, one could add, of an unresolved conflict *within* the individual. The fact that such an idea has been clinically confirmed does severe damage to Descartes' idea of pain and its modern counterparts. In the case of causalgia, post-herpetic pain (an excruciating nerve-pain following shingles), the body pains of the paraplegic or the phantom limb pain of the amputee, the nervous system activates itself in a desperate existential purpose of its own. Psychogenic pain – in the face, the lower back or wherever – creates bewildering problems of conversion and other psycho-semantics with which the bell-pull and the burglar alarm clearly cannot cope.

But what decisively buries Descartes model is the extreme relativity of the pain phenomenon. Whether it is the prick of a thorn, a hammer on the thumb or a child's stomach ache, the experience of pain varies not only according to the culture and circumstances in which a person grows up, but also as between members of the same culture according to the mind's participation – conscious or otherwise – in the process.

One of my first memories of watching football was the 1956 televised Cup Final between Manchester City and Birmingham. Towards the end of the game the City keeper Bert Trautmann leapt for a difficult high cross and, cannoning off another player, crunched sickeningly into the goal upright. After a delay while he received the usual baptism with bucket and sponge, Trautmann resumed his place on the goal line, playing with distinction until the final whistle. Only three days later, after X-rays were taken, was it discovered that for ten minutes he had jumped, caught and flung himself about the goal-mouth with a broken neck. Trautmann's heroism caused a sensation. How had he done it?

An answer can be found in the experience of troops wounded in war. During the Second World War, H. K. Beecher, a MASH surgeon, was amazed to encounter two out of three very seriously wounded men who either felt no pain at all, or else had so little that they refused morphine. Beecher reported that this effect, which he observed in 65 per cent of soldiers, lasted for hours or even days, but when he looked for the same thing in civilians after major traumatic surgery, he found that only 20 per cent had no pain. Very similar levels of anaesthesia were later experienced amongst Israeli troops who lost limbs in battle during the Yom Kippur War. Bert Trautmann was in part responding to similar circumstances: with the game afoot, the high excitement and an 'England expects' team mentality, his system was so hyped up that he had no use for pain.

There is a cultural element mixed into all this, because individual societies – and individuals within them – each produce different responses to Nelson's Trafalgar signal. In general the relationship between how the pain is *perceived*, how it is *felt* and how it is *shown* are to some extent determined by upbringing and origin – and to a very large extent by a person's whole experience.

To analyse fully Trautmann's feat you would need to know that he was German-born and had been a prisoner-of-war who chose to remain in Britain after the war and marry a Lancashire girl. It might also be worth knowing that only a month before his dramatic Cup Final he had been voted Footballer of the Year. His upbringing, personality, status and the unusual path which brought him to Wembley must all have played their part in enabling him to deny the pain and play on.

In international football it is noticeable that players from some countries show the pain of a kick or a fall more uninhibitedly – some might say, histrionically – than those from others. But they are not necessarily acting. It was shown in 1952[5] that there is wide variation in the thresholds of pain perception between different ethnic groups, even though *sensation* thresholds remain identical across all groups. In other words, although all people are equally aware of a given stimulus, some are more likely than others to regard it as more painful and to react accordingly. In the 1952 study, people of northern European and of Mediterranean origin were compared. Each had a part of the skin exposed to a low level of radiated heat, which was gradually turned up until the subject announced that it hurt. The Mediterranean individuals consistently reported pain earlier than the northern Europeans: a finding which is, of course, in line with our idea of the 'latin' temperament, in which emotions are expressed more easily and forcefully than by the more reserved 'northern' temperament.

The knowledge that different groups may have different pain thresholds can give some spurious legitimization to racial prejudice. A journalist, Amrit Wilson, was once told by a group of doctors that, 'The pain threshold for Asians is half that of Caucasians – they complain twice as much for half the reason – they come with minor symptoms'.[6] Even if the claim of such a dramatic difference between the pain thresholds of Asians and whites could be substantiated – and I know of no such trial – the racism of the remark would stand, since the significance of the pain symptom is precisely how much it is perceived. People with lower thresholds of pain perception need to be treated with more, not less, attentiveness, because this *perception* of pain is of course the pain itself. Pain does not exist unless and until it is perceived or in other words *felt*. And how is the feeling of pain related to its *expression*? As this is such a subjective variable and cultural matter, it is a source of much potential scientific embarrassment.

Pain 'behaviour'

No science extends a particularly warm welcome to subjectivity, and since medical science very often prefers to masquerade as a 'hard' science it does not like to play with flabby variables such as 'personality' and 'upbringing' either. Yet, in the realm of pain at least, it has by its own efforts accumulated so much evidence for these factors that they cannot be ignored. Medicine today has therefore sought refuge in behaviourism, the most stone-faced of the schools of psychology. Take as an example *The Lancet's* leading article on 4 January 1986, entitled 'Learned Pain Behaviour'. The article's thrust is to separate 'appropriate' from 'inappropriate' pain – a discrimination which is left to the physician's clinical judgement following a physical examination of the patient. Appropriate pain is from any approved organic source, susceptible to clinical measurement. Inappropriate pain is explained in strict behavioural terms:

> If expressions of pain produce sympathetic attention (or any other desired reaction) from someone important to the victim and close at hand, this will encourage further complaints of pain in the presence of the same person. Complaints may also enable the victim to avoid other unpleasant activities, thus further indirectly rewarding the sick role. Behaviours that are compatible with being well are not rewarded and so tend to be extinguished. Often an over-solicitous parent or spouse may be encouraging this development – a syndrome termed operant or learned pain behaviour.

The implication from this is that learned pain is somehow less valid than organic pain, and that a doctor should be on the lookout for certain 'warning signs from the history', including 'improbable descriptions of the pain – for example "whole leg pain" – using affective words like "sickening" and "blinding" to describe it, progression of the extent and the severity of the pain over time, and multiple treatments.' Nor is the patient's body language any less improbable or affective, since it tends

44

towards 'exaggerated facial expression of pain, abnormal posture, frequent grimacing and sighing, and rubbing of the affected parts.' So, according to this authority, inappropriate pain can be successfully unmasked if it is expressed in particularly gross or extreme ways.

But this is ridiculous, for pain can be the most gross and extreme experience any of us is called upon to suffer. As far as vocabulary goes, 'sickening' and 'blinding' are legitimate and frequent enough descriptions of pain to be included, with eighty-two other 'affective' adjectives, in the questionnaire developed at McGill University, whose whole point is to provide some true measure of pain severity. As for the remarks about posture and grimace, we are getting close to a specialized case of Catch-22. Unless you can contain your expressions of pain within the doctor's assessment of 'reasonable' limits, you hardly qualify for help; if you *can* contain them, you hardly need to!

The behaviourist, at least, does have an explanation as to why the Spanish or Italian footballer rolls in agony, his face contorted, his hands clamped over the tightly flexed knee, while the West German – though he cannot help limping – shows no apparent emotion. The Spaniard's knee is just as likely (or as unlikely) to have 'real' pain as the German's, but his experience of it has more to do with his mother's knee (and what he learns there) than with his own. When it comes to applying this sort of analysis to the clinical setting, however, *The Lancet's* underlying tone comes close to the censorious, since it is speaking not of bruised half-backs but of patients who need sympathetic help. To regard them as claiming 'more pain than appears warranted from any pathological process that is present' comes close to implying they should 'pull themselves together'.

On this evidence, the treatment offered by this approach is equally bleak. The patient must be reprogrammed by 'changing the pain behaviour' and 'eliminating the rewards and substituting more active and constructive behaviours'. But we are warned ominously that 'only the well-motivated should be selected'.

But what about the hapless others – the unselected? 'The therapist is entitled to retire to the wings if no progress is possible', declares our arbiter. It is as if Jonathan Miller's 'pantomime of complaint' was, in fact, just that: a piece of theatre, whose actors can return to being 'normal' and 'themselves' as soon as the footlights are killed.

This approach has little appeal. To discriminate, as the behaviourist does, between appropriate and inappropriate hurting is pure sophistry: *a pain is a pain is a pain*. In any case, what neurology is now saying about pain *mechanism* is making it increasingly difficult to justify the distinction between one kind of pain, supposed to be properly organic, and another which is regarded as merely imaginary.

The pain gate

It is the relativity of pain which has so bedevilled scientific investigation. In particular, it has showed the neo-Cartesian burglar alarm to be of little more use than those rusty boxes attached to shop premises which ring unpredictably at all hours of the day and night. However, twenty years ago a theoretical breakthrough was made which revolutionized pain theory and, in the process, replaced the warning system of the burglar alarm with a pain *gate*.

Even after twenty years, the 'pain control gate' is still a medical guess. In order to understand how it was arrived at by two neurologists, in collaboration though on different sides of the Atlantic, we need to look back at our simplified explanation of nerve action and complicate it slightly.

It is important to note that each message-receiving cell – each one in the line of dominoes – is hooked up to many message-sending cells simultaneously. Numerous synapses cover the cell body and these receive in their neurotransmitters at different frequencies. Inputs have different effects, too. They are not all designed to *stimulate* action; some *inhibit* action. So whether the receiving cell itself fires in its turn, or remains 'silent', depends upon the weight of opinion from the inputters – exactly as if a vote had taken place. If the ayes have it, then the whole process is repeated and the dominoes continue to drop. If not, then the weight against that domino is insufficient and the message never gets through. Once a cell has fired, it rests and cannot perform again for a 'refractory period' of a couple of thousandths of a second. This ensures that nerve impulses travel along a nerve fibre as one-way traffic only.

46

The firing of a cell is an 'all or nothing' affair, and the impulse it conveys is always the same strength. So the *intensity* of a stimulus can only be varied by the rapidity of impulses travelling along each neuron, and by the cumulative firepower of several nerves volleying together along the nerve pathways.

The pain gate theory suggests that the first pain signals reaching the brain trigger pain control messages from the brain down the spinal cord. The cord has some kind of control system, imagined to be like the River Thames flood barrier; the strength of painful messages along the afferent fibres push against this, while the brain's own downward messages adjust the barrier according to the circumstances. The degree of pain therefore depends not only on the size of the flood, but on the state of the gate, which means that if the system is working properly painful stimuli are *always* under the control of the brain – and so, by extension, the mind.

The 'gate' is of course an image, but it is a highly specific one suggesting a mechanical (though mentally controlled) process. As we have seen, mechanical analogies should be treated with suspicion in biology, but in this case it might be worth enquiring a little further. For instance, if this gate is closed, just what is it holding back? And if open, what exactly is it letting through? I have spoken of the 'messages' carried along the nervous system, but what is the medium for the *inhibition* of pain? What stops the nervous impulses from being interpreted as pain by the mind?

Natural opiates

Some possible answers to this have been suggested by investigations into a group of biochemicals, known collectively as the endorphins.

For instance it has been found that electrical stimulation of one area of the brain produces powerful analgesia all over the body. How does this analgesia work? One hypothesis was that by stimulating the brain in this way you release a chemical which works in much the same way as the opiates – opium, morphine, heroin. The theory was strengthened when it was found that the drug naxolone cancelled out this analgesia, for naxolone is also an antidote to the opiates.

Opium and its derivatives bind to certain sites on the cells of the central nervous system. The very existence of these 'opiate-receptor' sites is on the face of it a mystery, since opium is not found naturally in the body. However, the assumption is that the chemical structure of opium happens to resemble a naturally produced biochemical, and that these sites evolved in order to receive this chemical, not opium. Given the effect of opium, it is reasonable to suppose that the job of these natural materials is similar and entails the blocking of pain, a train of thought which has led to the discovery of the endorphins.

Endorphins are biochemicals of the type known as peptides. These are a part of the *output of the mind*; that is, they are expressed by the brain and form a bridge between mind and body across which the mind's messages to the body's cells are carried – such as, in this case, the message to block or mediate a specific source of pain. The endorphins' involvement in the regulation of pain, however, is only one of the 'homeostatic' regulations which the peptides carry out. They also mediate learning, appetite, body temperature, blood pressure and, perhaps, sleep.

Their analgesic effect naturally led to the hope that, by synthesizing endorphins, a safe morphine-like drug could be produced. Unfortunately, the endorphins proved to have all the side-effects of the opiates themselves: they depressed the appetite, caused constipation, confused the memory and interfered with learning ability. But most important of all, they produced euphoria and *addiction*. This seems to me to be a very important discovery which opens up all kinds of possibilities about, for instance, the nature of compulsive behaviours – such as gambling, violence, opera-going – not to mention the even wider subject of physical pleasure. It may also provide the clue to one of the great mysteries about pain: the strange area in which pain and pleasure merge.

The enjoyment of pain

The fact that some people seem to enjoy pain is decidedly awkward for mechanistic pain theories, and has been very rarely discussed by neurologists. Even pain gate exponents find masochism hard to explain since to them, even if pain is not identical with noxious input, it is at least a shadow thrown by it: pleasure ought to be another thing altogether.

But first we need to make a distinction between those who seek out pain because they want to suffer, and those who do so for fun. A glance through the psychological literature makes the former appear less freakish than the latter. Pain's primary association at deep levels is always with punishment, so that people who unconsciously believe they deserve to suffer will choose to live beside the high-road of pain. Mr K.'s personality was in this sense partly masochistic, finding expression in psychogenic symptoms. Another example was given to me by a British neurologist from his own casebook. I shall call her Mrs Brown.

THE CASE OF MRS BROWN

A patient in her seventies reported having severe facial pain every time she walked from her house into the open air. It sounded like *tic doloureux*, a very unpleasant form of neuralgia affecting the trigeminal nerve – the pathway of facial sensation – which can be triggered, for example, by sudden cold winds or washing the face in cold water. But Mrs Brown's cold water was of an entirely moral kind, as her specialist became aware when he delved more deeply into her history. He heard that she also felt her neuralgia in bed whenever Mr Brown, lying beside her, turned over and momentarily stopped snoring.

Mr Brown was a chronic invalid, with angina and a history of three serious heart attacks. She cared for him with all the devotion and forbearance of a nurse, but because she was also his wife she did not feel entitled to take time off. Any absence or inattention on her part might lead to his demise, as her facial malaise would unfailingly remind her. Even shopping expeditions were penalized by her draconian unconscious; merely to sleep might be judged a punishable indulgence.

Moral masochism

Not all unconscious masochists are prey to psychogenic physical pain. If the somatic side of things fails to come up with any adequate self-punishment – or perhaps because of some inherent temperamental preference – masochists may alternatively insert themselves into painful relationships with others – parents, spouses, children, employers – in order to suffer mentally. Freud called this 'moral masochism' and devoted rather more time to it than to the physical kind, presumably because he found it more common. However, Freud muddled his contribution to the psychopathology of masochism in mid-career when he started to link it to the death instinct which, according to him, was not a deviation but an integral part of the psyche of humanity as a whole.

Moral masochists want to be dominated, humiliated, enslaved but not physically hurt. Their motivation springs perhaps from having no general sense of their own worth, or from a deep-seated need to expiate some specific guilt.

Freud also described the phenomenon of accident proneness, whereby a person may unconsciously cause themselves to be injured or otherwise 'accidentally' embarrassed or humiliated. In serious cases of 'psychoneurosis', he says, 'there is a constantly lurking tendency to self-punishment, usually expressing itself in self-reproach, or contributing to the formation of a symptom, which skilfully makes use of an external situation.[7] In the opening volume of his *A Dance to the Music of Time*[8] the novelist Anthony Powell illustrates this in an incident which throws a life-long suspicion of moral masochism over the character of Kenneth Widmerpool. The captain of cricket, Budd, throws an over-ripe banana across a tea-shop, which unintentionally bursts in Widmerpool's face, knocking aside his spectacles and spilling a glass of lemonade over his clothes. As Budd apologizes, '. . . an absolute *slavish* look came into Widmerpool's face. "I don't mind at all, Budd. It doesn't matter in the least." . . . It was as if Widmerpool had experienced some secret and awful pleasure. He had taken off his spectacles and was wiping them, screwing up his eyes, round which there were still traces of banana. He began to blow on his glasses and to rub them with a great show of good cheer.' The unnaturalness of Widmerpool's response was strangely unsettling. 'The effect was not at all what might have been hoped. In fact all this heartiness threw the most appalling gloom over the shop.'

That Widmerpool actually *enjoys* the (mental) pain of being made to look ridiculous by the captain of cricket's banana-shy is a ghastly paradox, an unnatural fact which is so disturbing that it pre-empts the ridicule itself. This is as it should be. The confusion of categories which 'ought' to be separated – such as *pain* and *pleasure* – is always liable to evoke fear, since it violates our sense of order and so seems to threaten danger.[9] In its most exotic form, where deliberate pain is transformed into sexual pleasure, the masochistic tendency can become a terrible and shameful secret.

THE CASES OF TWO FAMOUS MEN

In some tragic cases, sexual pleasure becomes impossible unless associated with the receiving of pain – a condition for which the pejorative terms 'pervert' and 'deviant' seem quite inappropriate when one considers the innocent age at which the association is (randomly) formed. The following was the experience of an eighteenth-century Frenchman, resulting from the first use of physical punishment by his foster-mother, Mlle Lambercier, at the age of six or seven:

> I found in the pain, even in the disgrace, a mixture of sensuality which left me less afraid than desirous of experiencing it again from the same hand. No doubt some precocious sexual instinct was mingled with this feeling, for the same chastisement inflicted by her brother would not have seemed to me at all pleasant.

But if this was only a child's mild spanking, a more brutal instance is the following description by an Englishman of the whipping he received from Ottoman soldiers:

> To keep my mind in control I numbered the blows, but after twenty lost count, and could feel only the shapeless weight of pain, not tearing claws for which I was prepared, but a gradual cracking apart of my being by some too-great force whose waves rolled up my spine till they were pent within my brain. . . . At last when I was completely broken they seemed satisfied . . . I remembered the corporal kicking with his nailed boot to get me up . . . I remembered smiling idly at him, for a delicious warmth, probably sexual, was swelling through me.

These two autobiographers had distinguished and famous

51

public careers which stood at an ironical distance from the secret inner lives revealed here. The first is the great educator, liberal and non-authoritarian, Jean-Jacques Rousseau; the second the British *Boy's Own* hero, T. E. Lawrence.

For Rousseau, the Lambercier experience described in his *Autobiography* initiated a lifetime which in sexual terms was pathetically unfulfilled:

> To lie at the feet of an imperious mistress, to obey her commands, to ask her forgiveness – this seemed a sweet enjoyment, and the more my lively imagination heated my blood, the more I presented the appearance of a bashful lover. . . . I have never brought myself, even when on the most intimate terms, to ask a woman to grant me the only favour which was wanting. . . . It is easier to admit a crime than what is ridiculous and causes shame.'

But Lawrence's is the more pitiful case. During the twenties and thirties – the period when he buried himself successively in the ranks of the RAF, the Tank Corps and then again in the RAF – he arranged to receive numerous beatings from gullible young men who were persuaded that this and other discipline was prescribed (and paid for) by a vengeful and authoritarian uncle who, Lawrence said, was effectively blackmailing him and demanding these punishments as 'payment'. This fantasy figure, known as 'the Old Man', might have been recruited from the pages of Victorian flagellation pornography (alongside Miss Martinet and Lady Flaybum): a curiously childish invention for a man of such sophistication. But the Old Man provided an efficient and necessary objectification of Lawrence's need for pain, a role which presumably could not be satisfactorily filled by prostitutes. According to his brother, Lawrence's motive was not sexual release but sexual repression. 'He hated the thought of sex. He read any amount of Medieval literature about characters who had quelled sexual longings by beating, and that's what he did. I knew about it immediately after his death but, of course, said nothing. It's not a thing that people can easily understand'.[10] But quite apart from the question such an explanation begs – what kind of sexual longings did Lawrence seek to quell? – it can at best only amount to a half-truth: it does not deal with the evidence from *The Seven Pillars of Wisdom* about the 'delicious warmth, probably sexual' which he felt after the Turkish beating.

The technical term for the sexual use of pain is algolagnia. How does it arise? Firstly, a certain amount of violence and pain has always been associated with sex. Havelock Ellis bases his long and fascinating discussion of the subject on the idea that, while pleasure is there as an incentive to reproduce, pain is also involved since dominance and submission are necessarily a part of the copulation of mammals. Thus, he argues, a degree of algolagnia, passive and active, is necessary to evolution – what today we might call genetically determined.

Be that as it may – and it may not, according to post-feminist accounts of sexuality – pain is in the *Kama Sutra* and most of the other ancient sex manuals as a sexual technique. Accounts of sexual fantasy and pornography are shot through with torture, domination and cruelty. In certain individuals these factors become essential to sexual pleasure, as powerful as the sex drive itself, but they are not originally matters of choice.[11]

Sexual tastes, which in humans are as varied and colourful as Audubon's *Birds*, are formed early in life, often as a result of random associations. But this randomness is mediated by the personality of the individual and, indeed, of all the people involved. Every little boy who sees his mother nude except for her stiletto-heel shoes does not become a shoe fetishist. Much may depend on the mother and on the boy's psychological circumstances.

Nevertheless we know – from Pavlov and more modern behavioural psychologists – that animals can be conditioned into (apparently) welcoming pain, and that early *sexual* conditioning, especially if reinforced by the stress of fear or uncertainty, is the strongest and most lasting kind there is. Also there may well be a connection between the pleasure and addiction associated with synthesized endorphins, and the endorphin-release which accompanies the experience or expectation of pain. A final case history, that of an anonymous Englishman writing in the 1970s, pulls some of these strands together.

THE CASE OF Y

Described by his publisher as 'a well-known author and critic', Y. came from a sexually repressed chapel-going background. He was privately educated in a system which emphasized corporal discipline, as the English public schools have always done. A combination of this with his guilty bisexual feelings has meant that for long periods his life had been dominated by a 'secret strand' which he draws out with extraordinary frankness in his book.[12]

Just one of the fibres in the strand is his continued interest in flagellation, though this is not an exclusive sexual need:

> I usually associated it with boredom, unslaked sexual hunger and a fascination with pain in this particular form. An orgasm, especially a wholly satisfying heterosexual orgasm, is accompanied by pain. The point about both is that they are intense physical sensations. Boredom is a state in which we lack intense feelings, or feelings of any kind. A whipping, like a sexual experience, creates, at least for the time being, the feeling of being alive, rather than half dead.

If this seems tinged with post-rationalizing, Y.'s account of his self-beating carries the force of truth, of a burdensome pathos:

> One of the pleasures of beating myself was the feeling of tingling warmth which followed. Alas, it would disappear all too soon, perhaps because I didn't beat myself hard enough. I beat myself as hard and as long as I could stand. I would take perhaps a dozen, perhaps twenty or even more strokes according to how well and strong I felt. When it was over, and I had groaned and become breathless, I would enjoy looking at the marks in a mirror and feeling them with my hand. It was of course a sad self-hating business, serving only to heighten the loneliness of my situation. It was a secret, solitary *schadenfreude*, sterile and unsatisfying, since it led nowhere and produced no lasting satisfaction. The only thing to do was wait until I could stand it again.

Masochism may be exceedingly rare, or quite common: I intend no statement about how 'normal' or otherwise it might be. I have introduced the subject because there is no other phenomenon which shows more clearly the relativity of the pain experience, and the need to place it in the context of *meaning*. Sometimes this meaning has a moral dimension: it may express loss or the fear of loss; it may encode the experience of self-blame. The rider to this is that the medical treatment of pain (where treatment is deemed appropriate) demands moral understanding on the part of both doctor and patient. Most physicians would agree that, in a general way, understanding is required in the doctor-patient relationship. But to introduce a moral element into a clinic which is concerned with *physical* pathology is a surprising and often unwelcome intrusion for those brought up in the tradition of mechanistic medicine.

Yet Montaigne's remark which prefaces this chapter should not be taken as a conventional piety. Given the existence of such a moral dimension in pain, it makes good sense also as a piece of practical advice.

Chapter 3

Skin

*T*he human is the only mammal without a hide. Instead there is this naked indiscretion which we call our skin, betrayer even of secrets we do not know we have. It is regarded by some as the largest and, after the brain, the most versatile organ. But I cannot think of it as an 'organ'. The skin is too inextricably identified with the self, too much of a subject ever to feel convincingly like an object.

During one winter night when I was fourteen, something happened to my own skin. The next morning, pulling on some clothes in the school dormitory, my fingers brushed a roughish patch near my groin. I bent to look closer and saw that a scattering of raised islands had erupted on my lower abdomen. Each was covered with a thin white crust, which could be levered off with a fingernail to form a flake. Gingerly, I tried this, discovering a vivid red area underneath which was slightly moist though not bleeding.

My skin's history had been normal. A finger had sported a wart once, and one summer a verruca had for weeks clung grimly on to the sole of my foot, so that I was not allowed barefoot in the swimming bath. More recently, a few preliminary teenage pimples might have sprouted. But what I was looking at now I knew to be of unusual and sinister character. As soon as I got the chance, I checked my whole body surface and found similar eruptions behind both my knees and near the point of one elbow. Questions came, exposing my ignorance and fear with nagging relish. Was it a loathsome venereal disease, contracted from some infected lavatory seat? Would I suppurate and then rot by degrees, going slowly mad as (I had read) syphilitics do? The full weight of adolescent hypochondria bore down and I postponed any thought of the school doctor. Meanwhile, my patches stayed passive. Almost somnolently the white encrustations grew back whenever I picked them off, but otherwise the symptoms had no interesting sequels. They did not hurt; they only occasionally and slightly itched; at first, they neither enlarged nor increased in number.

But a week later there were more of them, this time on my back. Or had they been there all the time – inaccessible, mute and unnoticed? Perhaps this thing was on the move and soon I would have a galloping disease. I also had an idea that some of my original patches were getting larger. In panic I hurried at last to Dr Gray, who was kind but impassive and neutral as without hesitation he made his diagnosis. He added that I would be allowed to take my skin to a specialist in York. The disease, he said, was harmless and non-contagious, though its name sounded unpleasantly serpentine. When he franked the condition with a proper name – a word I had never even heard before – this rather eased my paranoid hypochondria, but not my curiosity. I hurried to the library and reached down *Black's Medical Dictionary*.

Psoriasis

'A chronic inflammatory process in the corium, the papillae of which become considerably lengthened and more vascular than usual, together with changes in the epidermis which cause a defect in the horny formation that naturally takes place on the surface, and results in an increased production of epidermal cells . . .'

When translated by the dermatologist in York, this meant that I had something wrong with the formation of cells in certain parts of my skin. Most of the epidermis, he told me, is the 'horny formation' referred to in *Black's*. Under the microscope our outer covering is not so very different in principle from an armadillo's: a layer of dead cells forms a protective outer coating, our scaly armour. But unlike the armadillo, these scales of ours are flimsy, flexible and quite invisible. Also, they continually fall and are renewed from below. The psoriatic, however, has the problem of an over-supply of new skin cells.

In certain coin-sized areas of the skin, the new cells are manufactured in the corium – the fibrous layer below the epidermis – at a crazy, unnecessary and irresponsible speed. Each square centimetre of normal skin produces 1,246 new cells from a total of 27,000 cells. Psoriatic skin has twice as many cells for the same area, yet every day produces 35,000 new ones! Hence the raised red islands on the skin, and the suddenly thick and visible horny layer flaking off and continuously replenished.

The specialist in York confirmed the gloomy prognosis of *Black's Dictionary*. 'There is no cure for the condition and the best that can be hoped for is that it can be kept under control.' The disease is very little understood. It comes and goes apparently at random, with the plaques forming and reforming either in the same or in different places. The processes and reasons for it are not known.

That was in the 1960s and there has been very little progress towards understanding the condition since then. In time, my psoriasis left the trunk and limbs and migrated north to the scalp, where it dug in under the hair and has been an intermittent nuisance ever since.

I am lucky. There are perhaps a million psoriatics in Britain, a minority of whom have much of their surface area affected and are so disfigured that they become chronically depressed and housebound. Many more are secretive about the disease: they keep themselves to themselves, think of themselves as *apart*, and in such behaviour they unknowingly forge a link with their predecessors in the ancient world.

Unclean

And the Lord spake unto Moses and Aaron, saying, 'When a man shall have in the skin of his flesh a rising, scab, or bright spot, and it be in the skin of his flesh like the plague of leprosy; then he shall be brought unto Aaron the priest, or unto one of his sons the priests . . .'[1]

There seems to be some disagreement among biblical scholars as to whether all scriptural references to 'leprosy' refer to the same disease. The horrible degenerative condition which we know by that name was discovered by Hansen in 1872 to be caused by the *mycobacterium leprae*. That infection appears to have been endemic among the ancient peoples, although pathological examinations of mummified corpses from the tombs of ancient Egypt have yielded not a single example of it. But this is probably the result of a taboo like that in semitic – and most other – cultures, or perhaps simply the fear of infection amongst the pharaoh's embalmers.

Hebrew scripture has left us a rich written account of unclean skin pathology. The Book of Leviticus takes the minutest pains to instruct a priest in the diagnosis of what (in the English) it calls 'leprosy', but the criteria could apply equally to various non-contagious skin diseases, psoriasis being a prominent possibility. The Hebrew word *tsaraath*, which in the Bible is normally translated as 'leper', was probably intended to cover a wider range of complaints. In any case, *tsaraath* is of interesting origin, telling us much about what was meant by 'unclean' in the ancient world. It is related to *tsar*, which means 'anguish, affliction, distress, almost in the modern sense of angst'.[2] This means that the sickness was thought to be of moral origin, coming out of spiritual neglect and despair – a psychic not an organic problem. This reading agrees with anthropologists such as Mary Douglas who have argued that the concept of uncleanness has nothing whatever to do with health in its modern sense of *hygiene* and everything to do with its original sense: *wholeness*. We shall meet these ideas again later on.

Unlike *tsaraath*, our own word *leper* is entirely empirical, but it is just as likely to lead to confusion. It comes from the Greek *lepis*, 'a scale', so it is primarily a descriptive term; a leper is simply 'a scaly one'. Thus even in ancient Greece, and perhaps in Medieval times, many a scaly but harmless psoriatic must have found himself posted without ceremony to the local leper colony.

The association of disfiguring skin diseases with moral degeneration and uncleanness has persisted into our own times. Attempts to keep lepers apart were not necessarily to do with *disease* transmission, but with *moral* pollution. The advent of the 'germ theory' did not replace this, but reinforced it. The last leper colony in Europe, the two-mile-long Greek island of Spinalonga off Crete, was inhabited by lepers until 1957. It was a place symbolic of rejection and despair, of the same angst shared by Moses and Naaman and Lazarus the beggar in Christ's parable: lepers all. Yet it was no ancient institution, but founded in this century. In the 1940s medical discoveries had made the disease relatively harmless, but only gradually was moral disgust of the 'whole' – the hale/the not-eaten-away – for the 'subhuman' leper finally defeated. During the wartime German occupation of Crete, the superstitious Nazis avoided the place, ignoring the strategic significance of the island. They never landed there and did their best to prevent supplies of food reaching the colony. Their attentions were confined to taking pot-shots at the resident lepers from boats.

This glance at leprosy is not a digression. The disease's moral dimension, whereby a person is seen not as a leprosy *sufferer* but as a *leper*, is more or less present in all disease, for all disease is invested to some extent with morally symbolic significance. There is a tendency to assume that such significance only counts in diseases of unknown cause, and that it fades when a cause is identified. But, as the history of Spinalonga shows, the moral character assigned to leprosy was not explained away by the discovery of the *mycobacterium leprae*. It is not therefore the mystery of a disease, but its frequency and its visibility which gives it social and moral weight. We can see this clearly in the history of plagues and infections – including, in our own day, the developing threat of AIDS. Knowledge of the virus or micro-organism which causes (or rather triggers) an epidemic is, subjectively, not the salient fact about it. Of greater significance is how much we are forced to notice it, and assess our own lives in relation to it.

However, in discussing psoriasis, an understanding of leprosy is of additional interest. The fact that psoriatics were once mistaken for lepers may be the result of a superficial resemblance, but what if that resemblance is more than an unfortunate coincidence? What if it is a crucial element in the nature of the two conditions? Psoriasis may even appear as a kind of *imitation* of leprosy, or perhaps the two diseases are in some way existentially linked, like a pair of brothers, one malevolent and deadly, the other merely malevolent. Certainly, personal accounts by ordinary psoriatics repeatedly stress leper-like elements, particularly the shame and sense of separation which the condition engenders:

I pretended I didn't have it most of the time. If I saw anyone else with it the last thing I wanted to do was compare notes . . . . One's own distance is something one can't face in another person.

It wasn't something to talk about. Her mother had made her keep it hidden when it first came; she was about sixteen then.

I hated ME. I was trapped inside a body I didn't want. I wanted to live like other people, to be free to feel the sun and wind on my arms and body, to wear clothes I wanted to, to go to bed sweet-smelling . . .[4]

Control of psoriasis has traditionally relied on drugs – messy ointments like tar and dithranol, or else steroids such as cortisone. There is a relatively new treatment for severe cases which combines psoralen – a drug known to the ancient Egyptians – with exposure to ultra-violet light of the 'A' type. This 'PUVA' procedure has revolutionized the prospects for many sufferers, but it may have long-term side-effects, so PUVA is still not regarded as appropriate for mild sufferers, or for younger ones.

All these treatments can do something to inhibit the over-production of skin cells which creates psoriasis. But their action tells us nothing about how or why the disease exists.

As we have already seen, psoriasis is a disorder of cell growth and has this in common with cancer. The difference is instructive. Psoriasis exemplifies a *controlled* excess of cell production which, though it may wax and wane in the skin itself, cannot invade any other organ because its production is specialized to the manufacture of quite *normal* skin cells. By contrast, cancerous cell growth is *uncontrolled*, the cells are abnormal and tend to spread quickly and destructively beyond the organ initially affected. Some researchers hope that the dissimilar similarities will throw light on the cancer process.

As for the psoriasis process, the comparison with cancer has thrown up some intriguing questions. For three-quarters of a century, dermatologists have been plastering coal tar thickly on psoriatic plaques. We now know that tars are heavily carcinogenic, yet psoriatics under this treatment do not develop skin cancers. Why not? There seems to be some form of antipathy between the two cell disorders. Soviet research has found that if psoriatics develop cancer (from whatever cause) their psoriasis immediately clears up. Meanwhile doctors in Houston, Texas who are treating kidney tumours with alpha-interferon have noticed how interferon causes pre-exisitng psoriasis to flare up dramatically. Here is a summary of one such case.

A man had been diagnosed with psoriasis at the age of twenty-five and he lived with the condition for thirty-one years. But in 1979, when he was fifty-six, his skin completely and inexplicably cleared. Then, four years later, he had a cancerous kidney removed. Within four months, secondary deposits were found in the abdomen and lung and interferon treatment was started, at which point the patient's forgotten psoriasis made a dramatic and florid reappearance. For three months the interferon treatment continued and in parallel the psoriasis flourished, eventually covering 60 per cent of his skin. It only began to disappear when the physicians reluctantly concluded they could not save the patient, and discontinued the interferon injections. On the day the patient died of cancer, his skin was innocent of a single psoriatic blemish.

This link to interferon is extremely suggestive, since interferon – a natural product of the healthy body – is a component of the immune system. This will be explored in detail in Chapter 5, but for the moment it is enough to say that, if the immune system does indeed control psoriasis, then an *emotional* involvement becomes increasingly likely.

Family skin

Susceptibility to psoriasis – which is unique to humanity – is inherited and people without the inheritance are unable to suffer from the disease. But there is also a distance between the susceptibility and the fact. The disease does not strike all who might have it and, when it does, its timing – unlike many heritable conditions – is idiosyncratic. As the *British Medical Journal* noted of psoriasis in 1986: 'Our usual concept of a powerful genetic influence has to be stretched to accommodate a disease which may appear for the first time at the age of 108'.[5] Psoriatic skin must be 'switched on' and this can happen at virtually any age.

Just how the switch is thrown, and how the volume knob is controlled, are the moot points. Most standard textbooks admit ignorance, whilst mentioning diet and environment as possible contributors. Some include stress, but it is usually as a secondary trigger exacerbating the condition rather than causing the initial attack. Other dermatologists, disliking the attribution of physical illness to the mind, reverse the causation: the stress (*dis*tress) comes from the disfigurement and fall in self-esteem that go with the disease. My own experience and that of many, even most sufferers who are worse affected than myself, contradict this. There is no doubt that the disfigurement may mark the psyche, perhaps even more terribly than the skin. But the waxing and waning nature of psoriasis, like so many other skin diseases, often shadows the general pattern of emotional change. This makes it a family disease in the sense other than the genetic, for it arises so often from the emotional stew of home life.

From the emotions, it is but one step to the central mystery of psychology: the human personality. When manic-depressives also have psoriasis they find that their skin lesions perform a curious game of hide-and-seek with the psyche: when they are depressed, the psoriasis runs riot; when *they* run riot in a manic phase, the psoriasis slips shyly into remission. Is it possible that psoriasis is affected by purely mental states? In other words, is it a true *psychosomatic* disease? The introduction of this term provides a convenient moment to explore the philosophical problem of mind and matter.

Mind and matter

To the Medieval mind, there *was* no distinction between the spirit, the mind and the body. The vision then was of a smooth continuity from senseless lumpen matter up to pure spirit, so that nature appeared as a seamless progression from clod to God. Humanity, suspended midway between the two extremes, then became in our very nature a perfect fusion of mind and matter. In addition mind, thought and consciousness itself were essential *creative* principles. God was regarded as *thinking* creation all the time; if this process of thought ceased, so did creation. It was only the coming of Newtonian science that separated thought from the physical.

The conundrums of the 'mind/body' problem are ideal material for armchair philosophers, if sufficiently leisured. But for most of us they surface in the shape of odd fragmentary

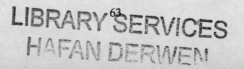

questions, raised in daily life. Everybody has been disturbed by *déjà vu*; many have had warts charmed away; some have had out-of-body or even near-death experiences, when the consciousness – the location of the 'self' – is felt to be detached from the body. What these have in common is the suggestion of difficulties in the continuity between matter and mind and the disruption of our normal expectations about cause and effect. A young woman I know works as a nanny; her job is the sole daytime charge of two small boys. One day one of the children fell on his head from a chair. There was a frozen moment of suspense, then the frightful wail of shock and pain which announced that he was all right. In that fractional second, the young nanny's own head throbbed in the very place where the child's skull had hit the ground. For the next twelve hours, she had a severe headache localized in that spot.

The practical account of pain given in the previous chapter is not very much help here, for if mind is immaterial, how can it reproduce subjectively the effects of a hard floor on someone else's rather less hard skull? The answer depends on the kind of thing we consider the mind to be – whether indeed it is a thing at all, immaterial or otherwise.

The BBC's *Brains Trust* radio programme frequently had as a panellist Professor C. E. M. Joad. He became famous for making all his answers turn on the qualification 'it depends on what you mean by the terms *money* and *evil*' or 'it all depends how you define *the law* and *an ass*'. Joad was often ridiculed for evading the question, but in fact it is a necessary quibble, since what we mean by things wholly determines what arguments we can use about them. By the term *mind*, protagonists in the mind/body debate have variously meant the soul, the reason, the emotions, the personality, and the awareness of one's own existence. In view of this, those who equate mind with the Christian notion of soul can plainly have only limited agreement with others identifying it with a Freudian psyche.

In the past, the physical location of the mind has also posed a problem. Today we are quite likely to feel that mind belongs to the brain as a whole, so it may come as a surprise that this has not been a universal concept. Aristotle thought the brain was a device rather like a car radiator, employing nasal mucus as a coolant fluid. For him, the higher faculties were seated lower down: soul and reason occupied the heart, and emotion the liver. William Harvey, who in many people's eyes was the first scientific doctor, thought the medium of mental effects was the blood.

However, finding the mind's location only becomes a project if you want to show that it has a physical reality. Objections to such an idea come from two diametrically opposed directions: those who believe that mind equals soul are obviously opposed to it. So, too, are strict materialists such as the philosopher Gilbert Ryle. He became famous – at around the same time as Joad, although on an altogether 'higher' plane – for trying to abolish the mind/body problem on the grounds that it is a 'logical category mistake'. Ryle's *Concept of Mind* makes mind just that: a concept, with no independent existence of the kind that matter has.

To me, Ryle stops at the point where the argument is getting interesting. He prepares the groundwork for a discussion by answering the Joad-type question about what *he* means by mind, and having asserted confidently that this is also how everyday language sees it – for Ryle, that was the only yardstick of reality – he leaves off. There are apparently no further implications.

Ryle's views have been influential not least because they give scientists an easy way out of the mind/body problem. Mind is irrelevant, they say, because logically it cannot be mentioned in the same context as the body. The body is a thing; the mind is only an *idea*. But what is an idea, if not a product of the mind?

A concept of mind which relegates it to irrelevance is actually harder, not easier, to understand than one which allows it an active role to play. This is especially true in the medical field. In the case of psoriasis, most people who develop the disease do so in their early teens, as I did. Obviously this is a time when the internal chemistry is changing. But so too are the individual's external relations and reactions with the social environment, in which the mind is both an observer and a participant. During puberty the combination of physical and social change creates a situation in which the mind is playing for immense stakes. These include the whole of the identity, of course, and the struggle to break with the emotional allegiances of childhood. But as well as these, the individual is under strong external pressure from peer groups, parents, teachers and from the adolescent's own developing understanding of the world and the future. It should be added that the individual plays a part, too, in creating pressures for others: status and responsibility are chips in the poker game.

It is now quite clear that during this period of life psychosomatic illness is especially common. One centre for adolescent medicine (appropriately enough in the pop music city of Nashville, Tennessee) has found, according to the *British Medical Journal*, 'that those patients with recurrent abdominal or chest pain for which no organic cause could be identified reported more stress than patients seen for routine check-ups, acute minor illness, stable chronic illness, or pain with a clinically diagnosed organic cause'.[6] Many of these 'life-event' stresses are necessary to the normal development of the individual's coping skills, but their effects are so complex and various that it is not unusual for young people to become neurotic, depressive, anorexic, anxious. They are, after all, living through unbalanced times, social and biochemical. That there are often 'psychosomatic' symptoms, and that a favourite site for these is on the skin, should cause no surprise. One of these symptoms, which we have all had, is blushing.

The blush

This has always been associated with embarrassed innocence, though physiologically it is closer to the effect (as in the song) of mud on a hippopotamus: it cools the blood. The body's main source of heat is from within, as a by-product of muscle work. A burst of exertion increases the temperature of the blood, which threatens the stability of man's inner climate. The blood vessels in the corium respond to this threat by dilating; in this way more blood is pushed to the body's outer surface, where it cools fastest, and incidentally, reddens the skin. The fact that blood vessels (particularly of the face, neck and upper chest) can dilate without increased internal heat is curious. Here the reddening of the skin is no longer a side-effect, it is material to the process.

Blushing is a response to the sudden perception of self-consciousness. It comes not from muscle-action but from mind-action; not from the threat of heat but from the threat of moral exposure. Its function is to send out a signal, to express an emotional state for other people to read, especially at times when appropriate words are difficult to find. Therefore, it is not surprising that it should particularly afflict adolescents with their conflicting, undisciplined emotions and chronically stumbling tongues.

This expressiveness of the blush is not, of course, consciously willed. It can be distressing because it reveals an inner state unwillingly, which also makes it interesting to the psycho-analyst since it is, in a sense, a communication from the unconscious mind itself. The analyst Paul Schilder gives us what may seem a surprising fact that 'blushing is, as is analyti-cally well known, a substitute for erection'.[7] Schilder's remark comes during his discussion of the case history of patient Mr S. L.

THE CASE OF MR S. L.

He is a thirty-one-year-old third son of an aggressive, unloving father and sexually repressed mother, who warned him as a child against showing himself naked. From an early age his sexual fantasies centred around the idea of being passive and 'feminine', but these were balanced by an intense admiration for 'positive masculinity'.

His obsessional self-consciousness was particularly acute sexually. He was frightened of asserting himself, afraid of being seen defecating amd mortally afraid of being seen with an erec-tion. In general, he intensely disliked his erections. Schilder's description continues:

As a child he was interested in telephones. He liked to play at telephones and telephoned to a friend across the street. He ident-ified himself with this girl. He did not want anybody to know about his masturbation. He is afraid of others knowing something about him . . .

When he masturbated, he felt that the masturbation would make his beard grow. Even at the time of his analysis he felt especially self-conscious when he was at the barber's. He was very much interested in his face. He thought that his nose was too long. . . . He felt that other people were looking at him and thought that he was inferior. He also felt that they were laughing at him. He could not talk but blushed and perspired. He would have liked to be a public orator. He admired people who came into contact with others and were able to talk freely. He would have liked to be a salesman, a buyer or an actor.[8]

This seems to me no different from what the great majority of teenagers feel at one time or another: self-consciousness, fear of sex, fascination with bodily change and fear of the same – even an interest in the possibilities of the telephone. The problem which took Mr S. L. along to the analyst was that, at thirty-one, his morbid fear of blushing and sweating still tormented him. And this is where Schilder makes the connection between a blush and an erection. Mr S. L., he believed, was a repressed exhibitionist who denied these impulses by transferring them to feelings about facial blushing. After all, the flow of blood into the face's vessels is a very similar process to that into the penis, and (potentially) even more visible than that is. Schilder says:

> It is remarkable that the face now became the centre of his body-image which attracted the attention of all the other people. It was the tool by which he brought the body-images of others nearer to himself. Everybody looked at him, saw him and gave him attention. This was the attention which he primarily wanted for his defecation and for his erection.[9]

Yet although the blush is more socially acceptable than the erection, unlike the latter it is quite impossible to conceal. In addition, once Mr S. L. had made the connection the association stuck and he became just as ashamed of his blushing as he was of his erections. Mr S. L. had solved one problem by lumbering himself with another.

Some readers will find this psychoanalytical correspondence between the flush of the cheeks and an erection ridiculous. But for me the great discovery of psychoanalysis is that the psyche is capable of recognizing and using metaphor – in dreams and in everyday life. Ever since Freud began analysing dreams, Freudian psychology had stressed the unconscious mind's tendency to work through imagery, especially sexual metaphors. The creator of a rival school, Carl Jung, held that the unconscious employs universal symbols and metaphors (mythical rather than sexual) as a matter of course, and that these are dynamically active in the mind. In his autobiography he described his conflicting emotions after the break with Freud in 1912:

> To the extent that I managed to translate the emotions into images – that is to say, to find the images which were concealed in the emotions – I was inwardly calmed and reassured. Had I left those images hidden in the emotions, I might have been torn to pieces by them.[10]

The ability of the mind to create and use *images* may turn out to be its fundamental and most mysterious process. Materialist psychology cannot admit that there is such a process, since it denies autonomous mental activity. At best, mental images would be 'epiphenomenal' – side-effects of electrical brain activity with no particular importance. Jung's defiant suggestion – in an age of militant behaviourism – is that the images come *before* the emotions, and that they are so potentially explosive they can even tear him (psychologically) apart.

If any of these psychoanalytical ideas are realistic, the unconscious mind is an active principle engaged in creating and communicating images and far from irrelevant to the physical status of the body. Some of these communications are internal, for example dreams, but others are meant to be read by the world at large and the skin is obviously an ideal canvas on which to write such messages.

The psychoanalyst George Groddeck was well aware of this:

> You know that, as a pupil of Schweninger's, I am still sought out now and then by patients with skin trouble, and among them there are always some who suffer from chronic irritating eruptions. In earlier days I took no particular notice when I heard them say, at some point or another, in describing their symptoms, that they had sensitive skin. But now I know that their eczema ceaselessly repeats the same assurance, only that it speaks more clearly, and also describes the type of sensitiveness. It says – at least I think I hear it, and the results seems to bear me out – 'See how my skin longs to be gently tickled. There is such charm in soft stroking, and no one strokes me. But understand me! Help me! How should I better express my desires than through the scratching I force upon myself?' This is pure exhibitionism in the realm of touching.[11]

One factor which perhaps makes skin so appropriate as a canvas for the psyche is that, in the embryo, the brain develops *from* it. Just a *week* or so after conception, the ball of cells destined to become a person is differentiated into just three types of cell, in three layers. At that point a 'neural plate' forms on a section of the embryo's *outer* layer, the embryonic skin, and this plate later rolls up and sinks inside the embryo to form the tube which will become the spinal cord and the brain. But the genesis of the brain emphasizes the close relationship between the body's outermost covering and its innermost mental processes.

The body's outermost covering is more than just a birthday wetsuit; it is the largest organ we possess and also the frontier through which we admit some substances and eject others. It is an organ of perception with an extensive range of modes and subtleties, from temperature to tickling. Finally, it is an organ of communication and a sexual organ. No wonder our psyche pays so much attention to it.

So I return, again, to the skin condition with which I started this chapter. Skin – apart from all the factors above – is most simply seen as a wall: *our* wall. When psoriasis starts, medicine speaks of its outward signs as *lesions*, or else of the *plaques*. I much prefer the latter. A plaque is something which we stick on a wall and with which we intend to tell the world something. Psoriasis likewise.

Nor need we resort to Vienna or Geneva to form this view. Dr R. H. Seville is a recently retired consultant dermatologist from Lancaster who has never been sure whether his speciality is best described as 'cutaneous medicine' or 'cutaneous psychiatry'. I shall cite from his book[12] just one of several case histories illustrating the appropriateness of the latter description.

THE CASE OF THE MIDDLE PRISONER

He knelt between two other prisoners, all three of them with their heads on execution blocks. His fellows were beheaded, but the sword never came down on his neck. Instead he went back to the prisoner-of-war camp to encourage the others in their efforts to rebuild the Thai railway. If they failed, they would all face the block. Extensive psoriasis developed within the week, and never cleared.

The whole episode was only discovered when he was being

treated thirty years later; he woke on the skin ward and had a major abreaction on finding a doctor from the Orient standing at his beside.

Nervous skin

There is a recognized group of skin conditions called the *neurodermatoses*, which to varying degrees – depending on which specialist you are talking to – are caused by emotional disturbance. Moreover, the severity and longevity of the symptoms are graded. A transient blush appears almost instantaneously and probably fades in a few minutes. *Rosacea* is the more persistent dilation of the blood vessels in the blush area, causing a lasting redness. It can ultimately involve enormous enlargement of the sebaceous glands, which in turn may lead to gross and deforming enlargement of the nose, an unfortunate symptom known politely as *rhinophyma* – or otherwise 'grog blossoms'. It has no causative connection with grog, although the characteristic appearance of the poor rosaceatic is often supposed to denote alcoholism. In fact, however, the emotional state which leads to one might also bring about the other.

Eczema, or *atopic* (as opposed to *contact*) *dermatitis* is the next neurodermatosis. Its appearance is highly unpredictable and unstable; it causes a strong itch and a slight rash which, however, often becomes angry and scabbed after scratching. Eczema has a strong association with allergy, but is also clearly linked to emotional states. People who are predisposed to have eczema, as well as asthma and hay fever, are called 'atopics'. They are an enormous group, about one-third of the population, and can be identified because they produce excess quantities of the antibody immunoglobulin E. Atopics do not necessarily ever show the symptoms of eczema, but are more likely to do so as children.

The whole subject of allergy, a disorder of immunity, will arise later in relation to the immune system. Part of the argument there will be that the mind – particularly through the brain's emotional centres – is deeply and necessarily involved in immune processes for better and, occasionally, for worse. This is regarded as a 'controversial' belief, which means that some medical scientists cannot quite come to terms with it.

However, most do go along with a link between mental (or at least emotional) states and specific allergies such as eczema.

Psoriasis has also been described sometimes as an allergy, and sufferers often relate its onset to specific foods such as chocolate. Actually, its process seems to be quite distinct from the disturbed immune response of an allergic attack, although like eczema it has been linked to emotional turmoil. In both cases, this is still a matter of debate between dermatologists. However, we have already noted that the interferons – which we have seen to be implicated in psoriasis – are part and parcel of the immune system. In itself, that suggests a pathway for emotions to affect the biochemistry of the condition. Yet I have seen few modern dermatology textbooks which make much of the stress connection; there may be a passing reference to the idea that it sometimes causes psoriatic exacerbations, but this is usually qualified by a denial that it can cause the onset of the disease. Such a view means, for instance, that the case of the Middle Prisoner must call for some explanation other than the obvious emotional one.

There is, however, a good deal of evidence to contradict the orthodox view. The list of clinical observers since the Second World War who have seen a connection between stressful events and psoriatic outbreaks is impressive.[13] Seville himself has put forward the view that 'first, severely felt, but suppressed emotional stress can lead to an outbreak of psoriasis within a month, and, second, clearance of the disorder can be related to the insight gained by the patient into the nature of the emotional trauma.' We have already discussed many of the reasons why the skin should become a 'target organ' for psychosomatic symptoms. What evidence does Seville himself add to the debate?

In his controlled trial[14] he used dithranol cream to clear the skin of 132 patients experiencing their first attack of psoriasis. He then asked them if they could recall major incidents of stress in the previous month – the period which he regards as the maximum incubation time. Sixty-one (46 per cent) did make such a recall. Twenty-four of these had been involved in traumatic family rows, 18 had had death or serious illness in the family, 12 were doing educational exams, there had been 6 accidents and 1 sexual assault. Of a control group consisting of patients going to their doctor with minor infections, only 10 per cent said they had undergone major stress in the previous four-week period. This difference is statistically significant and also indicates that the association between stress and psoriatic onset among Seville's patients was not accidental. That contradicts the conventional wisdom – which holds that stress is 'never' or 'rarely' involved in the initial onset of the disease (a view restated in a recent *British Medical Journal* review)[15].

Insight

Seville's investigation did not stop here. He took another very important step towards understanding the role of the mind in this and, by extension, other psychogenic symptoms. Pursuing the path of 'cutaneous psychiatry', he explored the nature of the stress with those patients who had recalled it and attempted to gauge their degree of insight. This turned out to be a highly significant quality, influencing their future chances of staying clear of the disease.

For Seville, insight meant 'self knowledge: that is, observation and appreciation by the patient of the significance of what has happened that upset them, resulting in understanding in depth, with acceptance of reality – the veneer of superficial recognition only evades real awareness'.[16] Of the sixty-one patients, just half were judged to have this kind of insight into the stressful events which had occurred, but what is important is that the insightful group had a *very much better chance of remaining without a relapse of symptoms*.

Fig. 2. *The effect of insight on time before relapse of psoriasis*[17]

No relapse after:	3 months	1 year	3 years
With insight (31):	31(100%)	29(93%)	23(74%)
No insight (30:)	14(47%)	10(33%)	6(20%)

Seville has here stepped across the normal boundary of his speciality. He has begun to speak of 'insight' in terms very like those of psychoanalyst Erik Erikson, when he describes the 'one single endeavour' of Freud's psychology – 'introspective honesty in the service of self-enlightenment'.[18] Few conventional medical scientists are so brave. Many will pay lip-service to – but will not truly embrace – the idea that subjective qualities can be harnessed in their work. Such a position would certainly prove fatal to systems of behaviourist medicine and psychology, which is still the dominant mode in science. Choice is the important element missing from a medical ideology of behaviourism: the choice to be healthy (whole) or to be ill (evil – 'exceeding limits' – coming to pieces). Insight – the path towards health, as Seville himself says – can be chosen or refused.

This choice is not necessarily between good and bad. In the essentially *tense* stability which is inherent in any biological system – its strength, but also its point of vulnerability – any change of state (from health to illness, or illness to illness) must involve a trade-off. One state might meet the needs of a particular moment; to move into a different one involves losing some advantages while gaining others. In any event, pathology plays an *active* role which insight alone can appreciate and weigh in the balance. John Updike has written of his own psoriasis: 'Psoriasis keeps you thinking. Strategies of concealment ramify and self-examination is endless. You are forced to the mirror again and again; psoriasis compels narcissism, if we suppose a Narcissus who did not like what he saw.'[19]

In the story *From the Journal of a Leper*[20] Updike sums up some of the points I have been trying to make. The disease is a powerful and active influence on events, ultimately becoming a pivot for the eponymous 'leper' to change his life. The leper is a Boston potter, creator of 'fanatic' blemishless pots: 'If the merest pimple of a captured dust mote reveal itself to my caress, I smash the bowl.' His 'leprosy' is not of course the genuine article, though he never gives us the 'twisty Greek name' by which it is known. However, the description is unmistakable: 'I am silvery, scaly. Puddles of flakes form wherever I rest my flesh. Each morning I vacuum my bed. My torture is skin-deep: there is no pain, not even itching; we lepers live a long time, and are ironically healthy in other respects. Lusty, though we are loathsome to love.'

As the story begins, the potter is in the hands of a dermatologist and about to undergo a course of PUVA treatment: 'internal medication straight from the ancient Egyptians will open me like a flower to lengthening doses of artificial light.' With growing excitement he describes the two-and-a-half months of treatment, by the end of which, 'I am beautiful. I keep unwrapping myself to be sure. Even on my shins leprosy has vanished. . . . The skin looks babyish, startled, disarmed: the well-known blankness of health.'

But his restoration carries with it a penalty:

> Carlotta says we should cool it. She has been seeing another man, a lay priest. . . . A worse blow falls when Himmelfahrer visits. He surveys my new work, pyramids of it, some of it still warm from the kiln, which I have enlarged. He appears disconsolate. . . . He says these are good pots, but not fanatic, that in today's highly competitive world you got to be fanatic to be even good.

The dealer, Himmelfahrer, agrees to buy the new batch only on condition that the potter goes back to his old 'fanatic' standards: 'I spurn him, of course. I see the plot. He and Carlotta are trying to make me again their own, the toy within the gilded cage of my disease. No more. I am free, as other men. I am whole.' He has made his choice. Freedom from disease also means freedom from art, and who is to say which has been the principal objective?

Psoriasis initially struck me as meaningless, a freak genetic accident. But far from being freakish, it is quite common; and far from being meaningless, I have found it full of meaning. Whatever the initial *significance* of my own mild case – which I now tend to regard as irretrievable except perhaps by an exhausting search for insight – the condition *changed* its meaning as I changed. So, too, with Updike. It moulded his personality, but it also might have been used by that personality for its own ends. Another sufferer who has written of the disease, television playwright Dennis Potter, has implied something similar. His own exceptionally severe psoriasis, the subject of *The Singing Detective*, has made him believe that 'whatever is in me that makes my illness severe is also in my work'.[21]

To the believer in biological mechanisms Potter's words can make no sense. In that perspective the pathology of a writer's skin and the character of his work belong in different logical categories and cannot in any way be yoked together. In this chapter I have tried to demonstrate that, just as all physical pathology has psychological consequences, so no physical disease is without some *meta*physical precursor.

=========== Chapter 4 ===========

Infertility

One of orthodox medicine's strongest impulses is to try to relieve the patient of responsibility. Hence doctors often accuse unorthodox approaches of loading patients down with liabilities they cannot bear, especially with guilt should their alternative treatment fail. Naturally, if the biomedical model is one of a faulty machine, then spiritual and psychological factors appear meaningless in any case. Even the patient's own feelings are treated as vacuous, and only of incidental interest, next to the main thrust of 'rational' physical treatment.

Yet since it can be caused, as we have already seen, by subjective mental states, physiological disease is not necessarily explicable in terms of reason and logic. Why is this fact regarded by orthodox medical specialists – and by patients, too – as such a threat? In this chapter I shall try to answer this question and examine in particular its relevance to one highly emotive specialism, the treatment of infertility.

An emotional onslaught on the idea of mind-caused organic disease is contained in an essay by the American writer Susan Sontag, called *Illness as Metaphor*. Sontag's is a passionate diatribe against the idea that the origin of a physical illness can be traced through its significant psychological (or cultural) meaning. For Sontag, science has rescued us from the personal meanings we used to give to such conditions as leprosy, TB and syphilis, and which we now give principally to cancer. All such meanings were and are lies, she says. Disease is either random or else the outcome of objective political and social conditions. Yet our imagination cannot be satisfied with this. We fear disease in proportion to our inability to understand it, hence we make emblems of evil from our most mysterious illnesses; in our own time, this means cancer particularly. In doing so, we yoke cancer to many of the moral weaknesses and discomforts we live with: emotional repression, sexual guilt and political deviance. Sontag sees the twentieth-century attitude to cancer as symbolic of our need for scapegoats and simplifications. Cancer becomes simplified to an almost fascist degree; it is:

a vehicle for the large insufficiencies of this culture, for our shallow attitude to death, for our anxieties about feeling, for our reckless improvident responses to our real 'problems of growth', for our inability to construct an advanced industrial society which properly regulates consumption, and for our justified fears of the increasingly violent course of history.

Sontag is saying that disease must be approached only in the light of cold rationality, to the exclusion of everything unscientific. In its ultimate logic, this is surely a heartless argument, capable of removing even the notions of suffering and sympathy from disease. It seems to confirm the view of Ian Suttie, the British psychoanalyst and author of an influential work *The Origins of Love and Hate*, that 'science itself represents a flight from tenderness'. Sontag appears to think that to explore the *meaning* of health and disease is to risk a dangerous simplification. Quite the reverse is true, as she should know. It is the reductionist, the one whose colours are nailed to the mast of pure objectivity, who takes that risk. For the pursuit of a frigid scientism can, in Suttie's words, amount to no more than 'a peculiarly sublimated form of intellectual "play" '.[1]

Yet the belief that the only truths are those which dispense with subjectivity is very satisfactory to scientific medicine. Science, too, prefers to see reality as free of subjectivity, a collection of *given facts* like the weather or an earthquake. The reasons are easy to guess. The subjective is whimsical and often fleeting; it is impossible to communicate in its entirety and very hard to break down into parts for analysis or discussion. This means that to investigate the subjective mind you must revise all previous limits and be prepared to grapple with imprecision and even absurdity.

The doctor's unwillingness to deal with the subjective mind is matched by an almost equal reluctance in the patient. There is plenty of evidence for such attitudes in the work of the sociologist Jocelyn Cornwell, who has made a detailed study of attitudes towards medicine and health in Bethnal Green, East

77

London.[2] The people Cornwell talked to – working-class people from a poor area – seemed at first extremely clear in their support of a 'medicalized' view of illness. Yet on closer examination, this turned out to be utterly misleading.

Public vs private ideas about medicine in Bethnal Green

Cornwell makes a distinction between two ways in which the people she interviewed speak about their experiences and opinions. One set of views is for public consumption, and strongly endorses medicine's objectification of illness and (in an area with severely impoverished health care provision) stresses people's right to efficient, scientific and clinically objective treatment. This public version is almost unanimous in the feeling that 'real' illness is an unavoidable hazard of life – either predetermined or accidental – and that stoicism is the only honourable response to it. Even where stress is mentioned, this is heavily generalized by using such phrases as 'the pace of modern life'. Cancer is regarded as an internal predisposition – 'everyone has got cancer inside them' – triggered by an external jolt or shock, because 'it just takes something to aggravate it'. However, people suspected of bringing illness on themselves are regarded as undeserving of sympathy: the absolute right to health care seems to extend only to those with 'real' illness who sought 'proper' medical attention.

Two other categories of illness are publicly recognized in Bethnal Green. 'Normal' illnesses are the everyday infections (flu, measles, chicken-pox) while 'health problems which are *not* illness' are the common chronic items of ill-health or internal discomfort, especially those associated with ageing. Such problems are not regarded as amenable to treatment, not in fact appropriate matters with which to bother the doctor. So to justify applying for medical help, you must establish the scientific credentials of the illness as 'real' or, at least, 'normal'. To qualify, it has to be something divorced from the self and *nothing to do with you*, for as Cornwell says, 'by establishing the "otherness" of the illness the person is able to prove that they are not personally responsible for it because it is something that falls within (and comes from) the province of medicine'.[3] These were Bethnal Green's public views.

But interviewed more confidentially, after Cornwell had won a degree of trust, a remarkable change occurred. The people of Bethnal Green now began to reveal a much more personal and private set of beliefs, which quite dissolved their previous moral distinction between true and false illness. Instead, ill-health emerged as a personal matter, and on no account 'something that could be separated from the person or the circumstances of their personal biography'.[4] These people were well able to lift the blanket of official medicalization, and to see that underneath health is highly complex and depends on the balance of many physical and mental factors, objective and subjective.

However, a final disturbing point must be emphasized: *these private views carry no weight*. Though more flexible and less schematic, private feelings about health and illness cannot overcome the deeply ingrained public dislike of personal responsibility in health. For example, Cornwell found nothing but contempt for the government's *Look After Yourself* campaign, which emphasized the need to live more healthily. Even the idea of giving up smoking was widely scorned. As Cornwell says, the scientific 'medicalization' of health had always stressed the 'otherness' of disease and the patient's helplessness. If the trend of public health policy is to *reverse* this trend it will be stolidly resisted, 'because by making individuals responsible for their diseases, it conflicts with their most fundamental attitudes and moral beliefs'. This means that the things working-class people in Bethnal Green say in public about health – assertions in perfect agreement with the Sontag line – are more durable, more 'fundamental' than their 'holistic' private intuitions; intuitions which people also believe, but keep to themselves. It is an extraordinary example of double-think or, in George Orwell's definition, 'the power of holding two contradictory beliefs in one's mind simultaneously, and accepting both of them'.

The double-think of *1984* was a state of mind necessary for survival in the extreme authoritarian society imagined in the novel, a society where 'Ignorance is Strength'. Some authoritarians of medicine also believe in this dictum; they desire not only to absolve patients of any responsibility for disease, but to deny them knowledge of it. However, there is double-think at both ends of the stethoscope. Many doctors lampoon the whole notion of the mind causing disease, at least within their own specialism, for they often cheerfully concede the possibility in organs or bodily systems which are not their concern. Such doctors, who are still in the large majority, at least in hospitals, much prefer 'their' portions of the body to stay firmly within mechanical biology, enabling them to maintain firm control of treatment. However, when it suits them – when perhaps the available technology fails to locate the cause of a complaint – the fall-back position is nevertheless often to invoke 'psychogenic' or 'functional' illness, and 'learned disease behaviour' – the very type of causation which, at other times, is regarded as laughable.

In the rest of this chapter I shall further explore this resistance to subjectivity by looking at the single specialism of infertility medicine. This deals with one of the most emotive of all medical conditions and we will find much confusion, on the part of both doctors and patients, about how to apply 'rationality' to it.

The curse of childlessness

In America, one couple in five has a fertility problem – meaning that they want to conceive but have no success within one year. The British figure is slightly lower, one couple in six being infertile in the first year of trying for a pregnancy (the year being a conventional medical yardstick). About half of these will conceive quite soon thereafter, leaving – in Britain – around 50,000 new cases of infertility in the clinics each year. It is conventionally estimated that in about 35 per cent of these the fault lies in the man, in 35 per cent it is with the woman and in the remaining 30 per cent it is with both partners.

Professor Ian Craft, head of infertility services at London's private Cromwell Hospital and one of a handful of surgeons who began performing *in vitro* fertilization almost as soon as the state of technology allowed, acknowledged the distressing extent of the problem when I interviewed him for a broadcast in 1982:

The lengths patients will go to are profound. Some of them have even attempted suicide because they haven't achieved their objective. Some of their marriages have broken up. Many are psychologically deranged. I think they have this feeling every time they have a period that it is, as was implied in days gone by, a curse upon them.

In Britain infertility investigations are carried out by gynaecologists, which means that in practice the condition is often seen as a particularly female problem. This is neither new nor surprising. According to the King James Bible, the Horseleach – shorthand in the 1500s for a person of bottomless greed – has two daughters, both of whom inherit their father's insatiability. One of these daughters is the Grave; the other is the Barren Womb. For women throughout history the second has seemed as full of horror as the first, for in many cultures the inability to breed can be a kind of extinguishment threatening to deprive a woman of her reason for being. If she does not find another role, it quickly turns her into a 'non-person'.

The infertility specialist Dr Robert Newill, in an article for *NACK* (journal of the British organization the National Association for the Childless),[5] wrote how 'obsessional' women patients often believe they are more expert than their doctors. One such woman had accused him of inconsistency 'in that I was saying the opposite of what I had written in some previous article. I tried to give an explanation but she became quite hysterical and, sobbing, screamed "Oh God! you are no use to anyone!" and slammed down the receiver. I doubt if any doctor could help this sad woman. She is the victim of her own personality.'

Men may be as deeply wounded as women by the knowledge that they are unlikely to have issue, but they are less vulnerable – at least as long as society continues to value a man according to his paid work rather than his fatherhood. A woman's motherhood, on the other hand, is still expected to take precedence over whatever else she does, and the inner conflict may be appalling if she then finds herself inwardly resisting this social (and psychological) destiny. Even so, for a man to be told 'your sperm is not up to scratch' can be a shattering blow – tantamount to challenging his sexual performance. Such feelings indicate the way in which our attitude to our own fertility is closely tied to our feelings about *ourselves*.

The perfectly commendable desire not to tread on the raw sensibilities of the patient, or perhaps the more cowardly motive of avoiding confrontation and embarrassment, means that doctors are often equivocal about the causes of a person's infertility. This is partly a matter of self-defence. Since most senior doctors are still male, they may find it hard to sympathize with the female patient struggling in the mire of her distress and frequently screaming in anger and hostility at *them*!

The doctor's perennial dilemma lies in how to regard the patient, whether as a client or a charitable object, and successful healers will always somehow manage to square this. But Newill's account exemplifies a doctor-patient relationship which has completely broken down, in circumstances which are the more painful because of the heightened emotional climate and the absence of 'real' illness.

One effect of the turbulence around this branch of medicine is that a diagnosis of 'psychological infertility' will be made only with the utmost reluctance. When it is, it probably signals that the physician has now washed his hands of the case. Before reaching this regrettable pass, however, every mechanical avenue is first explored. Giving patients a mechanical clearance is often claimed as necessary if the patient's suffering is to be minimized, but if this is the primary reason it does not succeed. The investigation of 'the plumbing' is grossly invasive of a couple's privacy and creates intense strain and anxiety. A woman undergoes endless internal probing and examination; a man must do humiliating things, such as masturbate to order when sperm samples are required, or spray his testicles with freezing water from a houseplant spray before intercourse. Simply having to perform coitus by the clock and the calendar month after month can do extraordinary damage to a previously loving physical relationship.

The fact that patients are willing to submit to several years of such investigation, in spite of not being ill in the conventional sense, testifies to the strength of the drive towards parenthood. That drive or imperative is in the mind as much as the body; it is charged with psychological and emotional significance so that, though people rationalize their desire to become parents, they cannot help revealing the extreme subjectivity of the impulse. In Naomi Pfeffer's and Anne Woollett's book *The Experience of Infertility*, the women interviewed give a wide variety of responses to the question, 'Why do you want children?': that it is expected by relatives and friends; that childlessness cuts you off from friends with children; that a baby offers an acceptable focus for feelings of tenderness and love; that parenthood is a rung on the ladder of growing up; that to conceive is an assertion of independence. What is striking is the clear connection of each of these answers with the security of the ego, the 'public self'. They show that in trying to become parents we are less likely to be motivated as in the past by a sense of inevitability, and much more by insecurity and the desire to win approval.

The birth control pioneer Margaret Sanger wrote that, 'No woman can call herself free until she can choose consciously whether or not she will become a mother'; although Sanger's remarks were intended to promote the rights of the *fertile* not to become pregnant, it is undoubtedly equally valid from the point of view of the *infertile*. But what if the woman – or for that matter the man – is inwardly divided, choosing with two parts of the mind two different courses of action: consciously seeking to have a child, unconsciously refusing the whole idea? The question is a commonplace in psychotherapy, but to pursue it further and ask whether the conflict can in itself block fertility is regarded as profoundly shocking.

Anne Woollett illustrated this shock when she responded to the *NACK* article by Dr Newill already quoted. She referred to 'the sometimes very heavy comments made by doctors in the newsletter [e.g. Newill's tirade about women's personalities making them infertile and their partners impotent]. It was because doctors present an account of infertility which is so different from what we heard from the people we interviewed that we felt it is so important to present a different view, as we did in our book'.[6]

And in that book, we are told that, 'there is no good evidence to support the idea of the emotional or psychological causation of infertility. Such diagnoses are based rather on the personal judgements or hunches of doctors who have no training in the systematic assessment of your personality or the quality of your relationship'.[7]

This is surely a very confused statement. The authors seem to be saying that there are no emotional-psychological precursors of infertility. If they are right, then of what possible relevance is it that the doctors are not *trained* in psychological assessment, since they should not be engaging in it in the first place? On the other hand, if such causation *does* exist, then the training of doctors becomes a matter of crucial importance.

The opposition to emotional ('psychosomatic') explanations is often more ideological than rational, and it is an ideology which itself can be highly emotional: a hot resentment at the suggestion that one's own self can be 'to blame' for an illness. We have seen the same resentment in Susan Sontag and in Bethnal Green, where the idea of personal responsibility is seen as oppressive. For rather less libertarian reasons, the medical establishment also opposes such causation. Here the notion of psychological causes – far from being a principle of authoritarian blaming – becomes a dangerously *liberal* idea, giving patients ideas above their station and preventing effective medical intervention. However, while infertility doctors hate employing psychological explanations, they cannot always do without them. So patients who are afraid that their infertility, instead of being 'real' may be 'all in the mind', are told they can virtually discount psychological and emotional factors. But the reassurance is given in terms which are quite likely to leave them even more uneasy than before.

For instance, in his recent book *Infertility: A Sympathetic Approach*, Dr Robert Winston of Hammersmith Hospital, London (who, like Professor Craft, has carried out IVF) produces the following arguments against emotional factors in infertility. If such factors were important, he suggests, young women – afraid as they are of getting pregnant – would find that their fear protected them from conceiving. Yet 'this never seems to reduce the disasters that we see'. Dr Winston is here knocking down a cardboard castle. The relationship between sexuality and emotion is not so laughably simple-minded. Emotions do not work an on/off fertility switch according to everyday circumstances; their interactions with the body's physical processes are infinitely more subtle, because they must take into account the wishes of the unconscious mind. Winston's argument only works if there is no unconscious.

Winston's second debating point tends to expose him even more. Rape, he says – by definition an event fraught with stress – is statistically more not less likely to result in pregnancy than any single act of 'normal' intercourse. Why should this be? Can the act of committing rape have some vitalizing effect on the sperm? Or perhaps there is an evolutionary reason why forcible sex increases a woman's fertility. These are not comfortable possibilities, particularly for anyone wishing to project 'a sympathetic approach'. But it is astonishing that Winston cannot see how his argument against the participation of mind in fertility is, in fact, an argument *for* it. If some psychological states make conception more likely, then the way is open for others to make it less so. Winston even admits that this can happen, but only in the case of one kind of stress. The stress of infertility itself, he states, may help to block a conception, though even this would be 'only to a tiny degree'. But again he does not see that once he has opened the floodgate even a crack, the whole of human emotion is apt to rush through and show that it, too, is a participant in the process.

The two sides – radical and traditional – of the ideological divide in medicine may well feel they cannot go on meeting like this. Yet clearly they have something in common – a hatred and fear of subjectivity, which is seen as an enemy of truth. Objectivity, for the Right, is the only reality and it is under this umbrella that they gather to find technical solutions that will put everything right. This of course is a fantasy, believed by no scientists except 'mad' ones. Yet in various ways the public is encouraged to swallow it, since the popular endorsement of the fantasy of high technology medicine brings cash flowing even more strongly into the most expensive, most 'established' areas of medical research.

If the financial dimension of scientific detachment is attractive to the traditional medical power-brokers, its political aspect is what beguiles some sections of the Left, for it lends credence to the notion of progress and the pursuit of an earthly millennium. I am conscious that this might appear as a distortion of the radical critique of establishment medicine, but unfortunately such criticisms are themselves sometimes distorted by internal contradictions. In their descriptions of the treatment of infertility, for example, the feminists Pfeffer and Woollett are certainly not happy with the way things are. They warn that infertility investigations take place inside the whale of technical medicine, a maddening and wearisome process which usually seems to be getting nowhere. 'Medicalization' is a serious problem, since it tends to degrade and depersonalize the patient.

Indeed, Pfeffer and Woollett go further than this and

recommend the use, in certain circumstances, of alternative practitioners. They illustrate the unorthodox approach as follows:

> Your hospital doctor may tell you that you are infertile because your Fallopian tubes are blocked. An alternative therapist takes these conditions to be symptoms of an underlying disorder which affects your whole body and not just your reproductive organs, and the cause of this disorder to lie outside your body in your way of life. In many respects his approach can seem more sympathetic as your childlessness is concerned with the quality of your life.[8]

This is a bare-faced contradiction of what has already been said against the existence of non-physical factors in infertility.

The reasons for infertility

Male infertility – conventionally responsible for a third of such cases – can be put down almost entirely to one of two problems. The first is simple impotence – the inability to sustain an erection long enough to complete intercourse and deliver sperm into the vagina. Of course, this is not 'simple' at all. Impotence may be a side-effect of a separate medical condition such as diabetes, but it is usually entirely psychogenic, arising from complicated and perhaps deep-seated neurosis. The usual treatment is by psychotherapy, although it is possible to induce an erection artificially by injecting the drugs Papaverine and Phentolamine directly into the penis.

The second type of male infertility derives from the sperm itself. Sperm may, very occasionally, be absent altogether from the semen; more commonly it is scanty or lacks vigour. The reason for such inadequate sperm can be difficult to determine; for obvious reasons it will not be primarily a hereditary problem. Aspects of the medical history, such as a previous severe attack of mumps after puberty, are among the possible physical causes. So are certain environmental influences, of which exposure to excessive radiation is a well-known example. In such cases the mind itself is no doubt less involved. However, the psychological aspects of many other risk factors cannot be questioned.

The use of marijuana, alcohol and tobacco is associated with low sperm count, as also are obesity, excessive exercise and having a stressful job. These are clearly also linked to particular psychological states. The list of risk factors also features several drugs prescribed for medical conditions which themselves can derive from the psyche. They include anti-depressants, drugs to lower blood pressure, sulphasalazine (used in the treatment of colitis), corticosteroids (illegally used by some athletes for body-building) and some of the cytotoxic drugs used against cancer. In all cases where these drugs are taken, there is some involvement by mental and personal factors.

The physiology of female infertility is rather more complex, because there are more biological processes to be affected. If no ovum is produced, this is the equivalent of the male's failure to produce sperm. But the ovum, even though it is healthy and fertilized, may have its passage into the womb blocked. Disease of the Fallopian tubes (through which the fertilized egg must travel) is therefore a common cause of infertility in women. It is very often a result of some infection (gonorrhoea used to be a major cause of damaged tubes) and infections, as we shall see, are no simple matter of physical cause-and-effect, but are closely tied to the emotions and the unconscious mind.

Another reason why a woman may be unable to become pregnant, or to sustain pregnancy, is disease of the uterus. Benign growths – fibroids or polyps – may distort the shape of the uterus and, perhaps in the same way as a coil or intra-uterine device, frustrate the proper development of an embryo. The cause of such growths is unknown, though fibroids are the most common tumours found in the human body and affect one in three women by the time they are forty.

The linked conditions of adenomyosis and endometriosis – where cells of the endometrium (the lining of the uterus) grow in inappropriate places such as the uterus wall, the Fallopian tubes and around the ovaries – may also be implicated in infertility. The reason for the migration of these cells from their allotted positions is a mystery and, except where the tubes are significantly narrowed, the precise role they play in infertility is unclear. But the disease is especially common in Europe and

North America, where some authorities think it affects as many as one in ten women.

The last area of physical investigation into a woman's infertility concentrates on whether the sperm is able to survive in the woman's body. This means examining the cervical mucus – the plug of more or less viscous material in her cervix which at times of ovulation becomes thinner and more copious, and through which the sperm must pass on its way from the vagina into the uterus. A post-coital test is performed (which must be within hours of intercourse), whereby the mucus is examined to see if it is compatible with the sperm. Some women produce antibodies which kill sperm; in other cases, the hormone balance of the woman is at fault and provides an unsuitable medium for the swimming sperm.

Some of these cases of male and female infertility have involved infection or antibody-production and, as we shall see in the next chapter, there is now known to be a psychological dimension to immunity, the system which deals (or fails to deal) with infection and which makes antibodies. Such a dimension is even more evident in the biochemical operations of the hormones, and since it is these which are at the root of the great majority of fertility problems, we must consider them in more detail.

The chemical telephone

Hormones are of incalculable importance to every aspect of reproduction. They stop and start all the various interconnected sub-routines of menstruation, sperm production, conception, embryo formation and so on. Even more fundamentally, they are what make males and females different, being responsible for the distribution of body hair, the growth of breasts and the other primary and secondary sexual characteristics.

In the body, hormones are extremely scanty chemical presences, so scanty that their identification has been a marathon task which in some cases, according to Gordon Rattray Taylor, has involved the processing of 500 tons of (presumably animal) brain tissue – equivalent to one-third of a million human-sized brains – just to obtain *one milligram* of natural hormone.[9]

It was through the increasing knowledge of hormones that

the biochemical control of fertility could be realized in the birth control pill. Today, through press coverage of *in vitro* fertilization and other 'miracle' medical technologies, few people are unaware of the enormous research which has gone into the study of hormones – and which is continuing, for our knowledge of hormone action is far from comprehensive.

The hormones are a communications system designed to relay orders. The release of some hormones activates processes (to do with growth and metabolism as well as reproduction), while others inhibit them. These messages going back and forth form *feedback* loops whose effect is to maintain discipline and stability in the body's internal environment. The endocrine organs which make the hormones are the users of this system which is like a military chain of command, with hierarchies of authority. The most important of the endocrine glands is the hypothalamus which, sitting in the mid-brain, operates as a kind of staff headquarters for most of the hormonal systems deployed around the body. The units with which it communicates down its chemical field telephone are the other endocrine glands such as the pancreas, adrenals, ovaries, testicles, stomach wall, thyroid, parathyroid and pituitary.

It does not speak to all these units directly, however. In its control of ovum and sperm production, for example, it can only order the relevant glands into action through a brigade headquarters in the pituitary, which lies in the brain near the hypothalamus. It does this in the form of *gonadotrophin release hormone* (GnRH). Receiving this hormone, the pituitary in turn feeds instructions down the line, using its own hormones, to the reproductive organs. In the male's case, the pituitary's *luteneizing hormone* (LH) passes on the order to the testes to make male sex hormones such as testosterone (which shape the body's characteristic male appearance and orientation), while its follicle-stimulating hormone (FSH) attends to sperm production. There is a continual traffic of hormonal 'orders' and acknowledgements along these lines which adjusts the levels of activity according to needs.

Thus fertility, or the correct functioning of the reproductive capacity, largely depends upon whether the correct chemical instructions are issued. The fountainhead of these instructions is the hypothalamus, and it is here that we should look for the link which couples reproductive status with the emotions.

Hypothalamus

Every St Valentine's card dutifully perpetuates the myth of the heart as the seat of emotion, but there is another centre with a much better claim. The heart, we know, is responsive to emotion because of the influence of the autonomic nervous system (ANS) – our repertoire of unconscious and automatic responses which adjust our physical state according to circumstances. But behind the heart's variable beat, behind the ANS which regulates it, is this tiny sliver of brain – the hypothalamus – which weight for weight must be reckoned the most influential four and a half grams of tissue in the body. As regulator of the ANS it looks after our body temperature, sleep pattern, appetite and thirst control, all of which are affected by emotion.

Brain mapping has helped to confirm this. The pioneer American physiologist Walter Cannon established that the emotional responses of animals remained intact even when the 'higher systems' of the brain are missing. Such primitive emotions undoubtedly originate from the deep centre of the brain (the 'fore-brain'), in the area known as the *limbic system*, consisting of the amygdala (the almond – because it is almond-shaped), the thalamus and hypothalamus which are both close by. If the hypothalamic area is stimulated electrically, fear and rage can be evoked – sometimes frighteningly. Patients unfortunate enough to have a tumour of the *thalamus* can produce a smile only on the opposite side of their face to the side of the tumour. When a monkey's amygdalae are removed, its behaviour changes profoundly; it becomes hyper-sexual and sheds inhibitions, handling snakes and eating meat as it would never normally do. There is complete loss of control over instinctual emotions.

The more complex of the *human* emotions, coupled as they are to the reasoning and cognitive ability of the brain cortex, must of course have a far more complicated origin. But they all contain elements of the primitive in them; they all refer back to the limbic system and so to the hypothalamus.[10]

Psychological infertility

It is believed that the average sperm count of American males has steadily decreased over the last two or three generations. At least one long-term study, into the male population of Florida, supports this belief. In the 1930s, when the research began, it was found that one man in twenty-five was sterile; the study indicates that the figure for today is one in five, a *five-fold* increase.[11] Even if we take account of increased pollution by chemicals and radiation, this is a remarkably disturbing change. On the basis of what has been said so far, the cause may be – if not wholly, then in part – social and psychological. So let us explore this further. The past forty years have been a period when the public perception of the man's ego-identity has undergone rapid revision. So have his sexual behaviour and the nature of his relationship to women. Is this a coincidence? What used to be called the Sex War – essentially a kind of private domestic guerrilla fighting – has developed into a more public campaign, fought out as much in the workplace and in the political arena as in the kitchen and the bedroom. There has been a simultaneous explosion in the rate of marriage break-down, with half the marriages in America and a third in Britain destined to end in divorce. This downgrading of marriage into, *de facto*, a temporary social and sexual convenience must have significant effects on attitudes towards parenthood. Finally, and especially in America, there has been a great increase in the consciousness of homosexuality and this, too, must have forced a great many to re-evaluate their idea of what it means to be male. Such widespread social and sexual pressures mean a higher rate of sexual insecurity in men, and since a man's ideas about his fertility are closely interconnected with his sexual identity, they may be at the root of the decline in sperm count. To prove this, a causal link between low sperm and lack of a positive sexual identity would have to be established, and this has yet to be done. However, the progressive inhibition of sperm production *has* been noted in some men undergoing infertility investigations – an indication that there could be a vicious circle involved in male fertility treatment.

There is every reason to expect that such social changes as I have described affect women's fertility, too. Like the man's sperm production, the woman's menstrual cycle is controlled by the coupled brain-glands the hypothalamus and the pituitary. Under stress the hypothalamus produces hormonal inhibition of FSH, the effect of which can be to extend the menstrual cycle for extremely long periods, and even apparently to stop normal production of ova altogether (amenorrhea). It is a matter of common experience that menstruation is affected by emotional pressures, but also that such effects vary from one individual to another. Among animals, it varies between species: some captive animals (such as the Giant Panda) have great difficulty in breeding normally, whilst others may become more fertile. It has been noticed, too, that even though their menstruation is initially normal, women married to infertile men sometimes develop serious menstrual disturbances if they undergo artificial insemination by donor.[12]

With characteristic thoroughness, Swedes have studied the entire female population of one of their major cities, Uppsala. This research conclusively demonstrated the correlation between psychological stress and the lack of menstrual periods in some women. It also showed that more underweight women have irregular or peculiar menstruation, which accords with the well-known fact that women athletes and anorexics normally have amenorrhea. In the case of anorexia, which I shall look at in more detail in a later chapter, it is reasonable to assume an emotional link on physiological grounds, since the hypothalamus is closely involved with the emotions and appetite control. However, the point to bear in mind is that stress is a subjective factor. What one woman or man experiences as a strain leading to chronic inner conflict may have no lasting effect on another. The key variable is the ability to *cope*.

Treating infertility

The most striking impression of the clinical treatment of infertility is that these psychological factors are almost completely excluded from serious consideration. If a hormonal deficiency or imbalance is diagnosed, attempts are made to correct it by the artificial stimulation of hormone production with such drugs as Clomiphene or the use of actual hormone, as in the 'fertility drug' Pergonal. This is a combination of LH and FSH extracted from the urine of menopausal women, which is rich in these hormones. It has the drawback that 25 per cent of Pergonal pregnancies are multiple, usually twins but occasionally triplets or even quads.

The condition of infertility is commonly approached as if it were a plumbing problem. In this case the invasive technique of laparoscopy looms large, an operation done under general anaesthetic and requiring a stay in hospital. The laparascope is a pencil-thin telescope with its own light source, through which the surgeon inspects the reproductive organs and hopes to diagnose the problem.

If the Fallopian tubes are deemed to be blocked, an attempt at micro-surgery may be made to cut out the blocked section and reconnect the tubes. However, *in-vitro* fertilization (IVF) – more widely but inaccurately known as the production of 'test-tube babies' – is now regarded as the most sophisticated way of dealing with blocked tubes. It is an extreme case of the research-based medical process, in which the patient's 'plumbing' is circumvented by the application of advanced biochemical knowledge. IVF enables conception to take place outside the body, first by stimulating egg-production with fertility drugs and then specially harvesting them by laparoscopy. Usually several eggs are fertilized (not in test-tubes but in a shallow Petri dish) and if they begin to grow, they are reimplanted in the uterus – though nowadays some are often kept back and frozen for possible later use.

It is not safe to assume that, once the embryo is inside the uterus, nature can take its course. Unconventional methods of conception outside the body mean that pregnancy-sustaining hormones necessary during the first weeks of the embryo's life are not produced naturally. These must be artificially supplied in a cocktail of hormones to sustain the developing embryo and prevent spontaneous abortion. Fertility clinics are still experimenting with different hormone regimes. At the Queen Victoria Medical Centre in Melbourne, Australia, which carried out the first implants of embryos formed from eggs provided not by the patient but by a donor, the patient receives two milligrams of oral oestradiol valerate and 100 milligrams of intra-muscular progesterone daily for the first nineteen weeks of pregnancy.

Such treatments are the logical procedures of allopathy, the process, described in Chapter 1, of introducing substances from outside to compensate for imbalances and deficiencies within the biology of the patient. Much of this is a question of trial and error, with the margins of error kept wide by the use of polypharmacy. It is not generally realized that IVF clinics tend to have their own hormone-protocols, for there is as yet no consensus on the best formulae. This element of hit-or-miss is disturbing enough; it is even more so when you know that the long-term effects of the allopathic administration of hormones and their mimics are a matter of speculation.

If the experience of the past is anything to go by, reassurances about the long-term safety of these hormones and fertility drugs are far from trustworthy. In the late 1940s a synthetic mimic of oestrogen called diethylstilboestrol (DES) began to be used to treat pregnant women at risk of miscarriage. Soon DES became the standard treatment across America for such patients, its safety unquestioned because no harm could be detected in the infertile women who received it. But tragically, as it turned out, those looking for harmful effects were looking in the wrong place. When the serious side-effects of DES did appear twenty years on, they were not found in the patients themselves but in their children.[13]

In the first place, daughters of mothers treated with DES were discovered to have a relatively high risk of vaginal cancer in their teens – as many as one and a half in every thousand. But much more common are the deformities of the reproductive organs which turned up in up to two-thirds of these daughters, making many of them even less fertile than their mothers had been. The sons also had a remarkable incidence of genital deformity, and one quarter had defective sperm.

The ironies of the story multiply: it was found as early as 1953 that the rate of miscarriage after DES was actually (slightly) *higher* than among patients not treated with the drug. This finding was ignored and new uses for DES were invented so that two to three million American women were eventually given the drug. Later, the long-term effects on these women themselves began to be seen. A study carried out at the Norris Cotton Cancer Center in Hanover, New Hampshire, found them to be up to 50 per cent more likely to develop breast cancer. The drug was not finally banned in the US until the early seventies. It was employed in France until 1977, and in parts of the Third World it is still used.

Such allopathic manipulation of the organism as the use of fertility drugs and IVF is reminiscent of the violence of Medieval and Renaissance medicine, where foreign substances and mechanical procedures were also used to try to supply the body's deficiencies. Nevertheless, such modes of treatment bring the doctor no closer to the cause of the original breakdown; they deal only with the symptoms, and that rather crudely. DES does mimic oestrogen, but it is quite different from it. It cannot 'speak' to the pituitary on the hormonal telephone, for instance. It can only override it, and in the process may do damage to many of the other functions of that vital gland, such as the control of the thyroid.

Yet if no psychological dimension is considered – and as we have noted, few infertility doctors are trained or equipped to do so – there must be obvious dangers. If infertility is in certain instances a defence against motherhood – or fatherhood, for that matter – then to break those defences by any of these means is potentially damaging to parents and child. And in such a situation, to bring about *multiple* births sounds downright irresponsible! Where fear of having a child is at the root of the difficulty, the answer is surely not in repairing or skirting round the pipework, nor in furnishing the hormones that the organism itself declines to produce, but in some form of psychotherapy. For such fear is rooted in the unconscious mind; as Groddeck said, 'If you hate your parent, you will fear your own child.'

So although IVF or hormone treatment is sometimes a success, leading to successful and joyful parenthood, its long-term consequences may be disastrous if the parent is not really ready for parenthood. John Harrison, the Australian psychotherapist, has written on this from his own clinical experience. He says that 'injunctions and early life-decisions' affect fertility, and he offers the case history of his patient Melissa as an example.[14]

THE CASE OF MELISSA

She was thirty years old and had been married for eight years. To please her husband, she had been trying unsuccessfully to conceive for most of that time. Her husband's sperm count was normal and no fault could be found in her own reproductive tract. However, she was not ovulating normally.

Her husband wanted children, but privately she had doubts about motherhood. It turned out that this derived from the experience of being violently resented by her own mother. Her father had loved his daughter extravagantly and although Melissa enjoyed this, she knew how her mother had felt betrayed by it. The mother's violent jealousy conditioned Melissa into believing this to be a universal consequence of parenthood, so understandably she feared conceiving a child of her own. She felt it would spoil her loving relationship with her husband and into the bargain wreck her life.

Harrison's psychotherapy convinced her that her parents' behaviour was by no means universal and need not be repeated in her own case. Her doctor must have known that his therapy was successful because Melissa's hormones began to flow normally again: 'Her body changed significantly over a period of six months. The somewhat girlish figure was replaced by a much fuller womanly sensuality, the type one associates with women who enjoy their sexuality immensely'. After an interval during which she decided to start using contraception – a clear indication to Harrison that she had begun to gain insight – Melissa conceived normally.

What strikes one most forcefully about this case is what it suggests about current fashions in infertility treatment. In the conventional infertility clinic, Melissa underwent every type of gynaecological screening, but her infertility was eventually diagnosed as 'idiopathic' or unexplained. Today she would quite likely be a candidate for IVF. That technique was of course originally developed for women with physically blocked tubes, but it is increasingly being used for idiopathic cases. IVF can even be used where a partner's sperm are too weak to enter the egg and fertilize it, in which case the egg is first exposed to an acid solution for 10-12 seconds and the outer protective layer is stripped away; it is then exposed to the sperm in the usual IVF procedure and, if it begins to grow, may be implanted in the uterus. This process was developed at Bourne Hall in Cambridge and announced by Dr Robert Edwards, the 'test-tube baby' pioneer, at a world conference on infertility in 1986.

The use of IVF for couples whose infertility is largely hormonal and may be due to psychological blocking is surely dangerous. There must be a risk to any child if its parents are not emotionally ready to adjust to their new status. This happens to many an offspring of *fertile* couples, of course, but to deliberately circumvent a natural defence system seems unnecessarily foolish.

However, even leaving aside psychological problems, there is room for serious concern over the IVF procedure. Had she actually received it, Melissa's IVF would have been expensive and statistically likely to disappoint. Even if the process does one day achieve pregnancy for every woman treated – 20-25 per cent is the best pregnancy-rate at the moment, although the number of live *births* is less – the question of long-term side-effects must remain. IVF can only happen because a great many different multiple combinations of drugs are used, both before and after conception. Bearing in mind that the unpleasant consequences of DES did not appear until the young adulthood of the children conceived under its influence, it must be an open question whether the use of hormone-cocktails such as the IVF procedure entails will be safe for the babies. Amidst all the press coverage and the scientific razzamatazz, this factor is rarely mentioned.

In the age of science, there is a natural impulse to resist moral interpretations of the body's behaviour. This is strengthened by the individual's fear of taking the blame for being in a poor state of health. Some supporters of the view that there is no psychological infertility will point out, rightly, that human reproduction works only under the control of our hormones.

In fact, this is the very reason why psychologically induced infertility is so possible. Like the endorphins mentioned in Chapter 2, hormones are physical entities, yet they are part of the *mind's* output. In computer terms they are software, disseminating the mind's instructions – and therefore its purposes – around the body.

These are not always, or even principally, rational instructions or conscious purposes. The brain's emotional centres are closely associated with the body's autoregulation, while the logic centres are not; the unconscious has a greater influence on hormonal processes than the conscious mind. In view of the obvious emotional content of the reproductive drive, I believe it is perverse and wasteful not to give more attention to the notion of psychological infertility, even though it is unfashion-able at the moment. As a corollary, it would be desirable to scale down the IVF programme.

Chapter 5

Immunity: conditioning and choice

'I know that you have disorder, though I hope not very formidable, independent of the mind, and that your complaints do not arise from the mere habit of complaining.'

So wrote the aged Dr Samuel Johnson on 31 August 1772 to John Taylor, upon hearing that his old friend was ill. Though no doctor of medicine, Johnson was, says Boswell, 'very fond of the study of physick', and appears to have acquired considerable expertise.[1] He had also, even in his private pronouncements, acquired an authority unique in English social history and by which he could speak for the England of his age. It was the age, certainly, of reason; but an age also which immediately preceded the triumph of scientific medical objectivity. So it was a reason informed by common sense rather than by any exclusive ideology of medicine.

Notice Johnson's double hope: that Taylor's disorder is neither *formidable*. i.e. *independent of the mind*, nor so trivial as to *arise from the mere habit of complaining*. Johnson was the great champion of reasonableness, so it is characteristic that he should be most fearful of diseases outside the mind's control, and most dismissive of those which come from mental laziness. We can take these to be fairly typical of the educated layman's ideas on disease in the period just before modern scientific medicine was established. Johnson's next sentence to Taylor is especially illuminating. 'Yet,' he says, 'there is no distemper, not in the highest degree acute, on which the mind has not some influence, and which is not better resisted by a cheerful than a gloomy temper.'

He should know. Not only had he been prey since the age of twenty to a battery of psychosomatic tics, convulsions and other complaints, but he suffered from acute depressive attacks during which, in Boswell's words, 'he felt himself overwhelmed with a horrible hypochondria, with perpetual irritation, fretfulness and impatience; and with a dejection, gloom and despair, which made existence misery. He was sometimes so languid and inefficient, that he could not distinguish the hour upon the church clock'.[2]

Johnson's intuitive prescription (for Taylor) of cheerfulness and mental distraction – advice he could not consistently apply to his own maladies – may have been something of an article of faith, but it is now being borne out by scientific investigations. Before explaining just how, we must first trace what Isaac Asimov has called 'a thrilling episode in modern medical science' – the discovery of immunity.

Immunity

Edward Jenner is widely regarded as having invented medical immunization in 1796. In an age when nearly everybody was pock-marked, Jenner admired the smooth skin of Gloucestershire milkmaids and, hypothesizing that their exposure to the harmless *cowpox* disease made them immune to smallpox, he tried deliberately infecting patients with pus from cowpox pustules – the process that is still called 'vaccination' (from the latin *vaccus*, a cow). In fact Jenner was merely refining and making safer a technique known to man for more than half a millennium.

It is certain that inoculation against smallpox – using pus from smallpox itself – has been practised in China since at least the early eleventh century, having supposedly been brought there by an itinerant Indian fakir. The earliest civilizations must have known that some diseases could only be contracted once in a lifetime, and that thereafter the victim – if he lived – would remain immune. A sharp-witted Far Eastern folk-physician, who must be regarded also as a heroic experimental scientist, anticipated Jenner by deliberately placing smallpox infection itself in the bloodstream of healthy people; he found, first, that a weakened type of the disease usually ensued and, second, that this gave full protection during future epidemics.

The technique spread along the caravan routes of Asia and North Africa and, according to the historian of plague William McNeill, acquired interesting ritual significance for the camel drivers, who would have had an obvious interest in becoming immunized:

> The person to be innoculated was viewed as 'buying' the disease, and to make the transaction effective, had to give ritual gifts to the person who performed the inoculation. The inoculation was made between thumb and forefinger so that the resulting pock-mark showed quite conspicuously, and identified the receiver as a sort of initiate ever after.[3]

However, it was not until the eighteenth century that Western medicine heard about it. In 1717 Lady Mary Wortley Montague – beauty, wit, friend of Alexander Pope and his circle – travelled East with her husband, the new British Ambassador to the Ottoman Empire. In Constantinople, the terminus of the longest possible caravan routes, both Western and Eastern medicine coexisted much as they do today in Delhi and Peking. The doctor at the British Embassy, one Maitland, had become convinced of the effectiveness of innoculation, which he had seen performed many times in the city. Lady Mary was also impressed and had her small son innoculated. When she returned home to champion Maitland's operation amongst her influential social circle, and even in the London popular press, the 'new' procedure aroused intense interest mixed with obloquy in about equal measure.

The enthusiasm came mainly from lay people only too well aware of the shortcomings of the medical establishment in dealing with a notoriously dangerous and disfiguring disease. Innoculation became a fashionable success overnight when Princess Caroline, wife of the future George II, took an interest – not the last time royalty would patronize heterodox medical treatment – and in 1722 had two infant princesses innoculated. Meanwhile, most doctors and many clergy denounced it as unnatural. One doctor wrote out of the apoplexy of a professional whose expertise is being side-stepped:

Posterity perhaps will scarcely be brought to believe, that an Experiment practised only by a few *Ignorant Women* amongst an illiterate and unthinking People, shou'd on a sudden, and upon slender Experience, so far obtain in one of the Politest Nations in the world as to be receiv'd into the *Royal Palace*.[4]

The few ignorant women had in fact planted the seed of a medical revolution, though its flowers would not open for another 150 years. This revolution was 'the germ theory.'

The germ theory

The word 'theory', we feel, ought properly to evoke a degree of uncertainty, even of mystery. So today there is something quaint about 'the germ *theory*': it has passed so completely into common doctrine that to use the phrase is like talking about 'the round-earth theory'. Yet in living memory it was controversial: George Bernard Shaw disliked it, satirized it in his play *The Doctor's Dilemma* and recommended people to consult only septuagenarian physicians, in other words those old enough to have been trained *before* the germ theory was universally adopted. Yet for most medical men the germ theory, even before any effective antibiotics were actually developed, offered an enemy to aim at in a war that had dragged on for millions of years: this was the war against plague, which after all had been one of the Four Horsemen of the Apocalypse.

The horror of plagues throughout history has been real enough and by no means the product of imagination. Yet the panic and fear which they inspired must nevertheless have frequently prolonged, enhanced or even, as we shall see, hysterically simulated them. Plagues have given man so much to think about that he has very frequently stopped thinking altogether and taken leave of his senses. The stress of the fourteenth-century Black Death was so great that it provoked extraordinary outbreaks of bizarre behaviour on a mass scale. Gangs of itinerant flagellants processed along the highways of Europe in states of ecstatic frenzy as they lashed themselves, and each other, with whips and tawses. In the 1665 outbreak of bubonic plague in London, people adopted quite irrational and dangerous beliefs; for instance that syphilis was protective against bubonic plague, hence in the plague year prostitution – with charnel-housing – became one of the few thriving trades.

Quite apart from its killing power, the moral significance of plague has done much to inspire these imaginative horrors. Many of the plagues chronicled in the Bible and by the early Greek historians had a virulence and significance which surprises us today, perhaps because the pathogens which caused them were then still vigorous newcomers. The Athenian infection of 430 BC (which may have been scarlet fever) not only halved the population and killed the city's indispensable leader Pericles, it brought an end to the golden age of Hellenic civilization. In metropolitan Rome, too, despite the outstandingly hygienic urban conditions, the city was ravaged by rampant infections – malaria, anthrax and many other pestilences whose identities can only be guessed. Rome suffered particularly because it was the hub of a vast military and trading system along whose roads and shipping lanes microbial disease was hosted and hoisted speedily within the bodies of troops and travellers – in the end, inevitably, to Rome itself. The plagues of AD 164–89, from which even Galen fled, reached mortality figures of 2,000 a day. In AD 542 in Constantinople (the 'new Rome') the Plague of Justinian – almost certainly bubonic – was even more devastating, reaching mortality equivalent to a Hiroshima every six days. In our own time we have yet to fully appreciate the full potential for mass mortality from AIDS, but unless checked it now seems likely by the end of the century to rank with some of the worst epidemics. Even without the intervention of unconscious mind, these are events massively charged with moral and historical significance.

By reducing morale and manpower in population and administrative centres where their killing power is most concentrated, such plagues have undoubtedly prompted the downfall of political and social systems. If it were needed, further evidence for the terrible moral destructiveness of infectious diseases is provided by the catastrophic typhus and cholera outbreaks of the nineteenth century and the influenza pandemic of 1918–19; the latter killed twenty million in two years – twice as many as had died during the previous four years of the First World War. But if people in the last three thousand years of European history have had a common experience of pestilence, and have in addition been able to some extent to distinguish its various forms, they have historically been grossly at odds over the means of transmission.

The possibility that the cause of plagues might be the activity of tiny organisms was not proved until Pasteur's time, though he did not initiate the doctrine any more than Jenner invented inoculation. It had been hypothesized since ancient times that plagues could spread by touch, or at least by somehow hopping between people. But since nothing could be seen of this, it remained one of several competing pieces of guesswork. Hippocrates, who was preoccupied with the uncontagious malaria, preferred to believe that putrescent organic matter gave off a disease *miasma* and that this was capable of infecting the whole climate of an area (*mala aria* meaning bad air in Italian). Galen, describing fevers, has nothing to say about contagion but speaks only in terms of unbalanced humours.

In the Renaissance, when people began to look for *mechanisms* of dysfunction in the bodily machine, the idea of miasmas was still current. In 1546, however, a doctor of Verona named Girolamo Frascatoro published his *On Contagion*, which for the first time elaborated a complete theory of disease transmission whereby 'seeds' of illnesses could be passed on in three ways: given by touch (like a relay-runner's baton); carried on some object being handled by successive people; or projected through the air. We perpetuate these categories in our language when we talk about *passing on* a disease, *picking up* an infection and *catching* a cold.

Gradually the seed theory became a germ theory involving a belief in organisms that were too small to be seen. This very slowly gained ground and resulted in a system of quarantine being applied throughout the Mediterranean ports. When, for instance, Lady Mary Wortley Montague landed at Genoa on her way back from Turkey in 1718, she was required to stay for ten days with the British consul before proceeding to England overland. According to her biographer, 'Lady Mary was allowed to receive visitors, but a noble Genoese kept watch to see that they did not touch her'.[5] Yet the definitive link between microscopic life-forms and disease was not made until much later when it became possible to isolate individual microbes, to grow pure strains of them and to develop dyes to stain them for microscopic identification. So it was not until the late nineteenth century that Pasteur and Koch founded modern bacteriology and opened the way for today's widespread use of vaccines and antibiotic drugs.

The effects of these techniques on general mortality rates and life expectancy are hotly disputed, but their ability to knock out *specific* diseases has been dramatic and undisputed; the eradication of the smallpox virus from the world has been one of the greatest ever triumphs of medicine and it was made possible by the germ theory in action.

But no sooner had he gone into action than the scientist was forced to confront a further problem. The great ambition of science is, as ever, to establish the laws of nature. So if you heat ice, it must melt; if you drop a stone, it must fall. Equally, of biology, you try to lay bare the irreducible principles by which the great soft machine of life ticks over. So following the germ theory, if you expose people to the bacterium *salmonella typhi* they must develop typhoid, and if to *vibrio cholerae* they must go down with cholera. These organisms cause those diseases, and that was that.

But unfortunately it was *not*, as an exploit by the Bavarian scientist Max von Pettenkofer showed in 1892.

Pettenkofer's challenge

Clearly something of a Professor Challenger, Pettenkofer snorted with derision when he heard of Robert Koch's claim to have discovered a microbial cause for cholera. He then performed a daring refutation of the claim. Obtaining from Koch a sample of his bacillus (cultured from a fatal case), he stirred a good quantity of the microbe into a glass beaker of water and with a defiant cry of 'Skol!' he drank it down.

Pettenkofer suffered no worse after-effects than mild diarrhoea, though his stools were later found to be alive with the *vibrio cholerae*. Other investigators repeated his intrepid experiment, also with success.

So why do infections attack some people while others equally exposed to them remain unscathed? It has been observed, for example, that in severe epidemics cholera hits young adults in greater numbers than children or the elderly. This is an utterly unexpected observation, since we tend to think of the very young and the very old as the most delicate groups. But, as pointed out by the doctor Albert Simeons – who had first-hand experience of epidemic tropical diseases – in the midst of all the fear and panic of a rip-roaring *epidemic* these sections of the population have a distinct advantage: either they know less of what is going on, or they are less concerned about it. It is those in the prime of life who most fear death.[6]

Simeons even sketched a possible mechanism of protection. The cholera vibrio – again to the layman's suprise – is normally efficiently killed by the stomach's high secretions of acid. Only under conditions of reduced acidity can it survive long enough to reach the more hospitable intestine, where it can thrive and wreak its havoc. And how does reduced acidity come about? 'The one thing that stops the flow of acid in the stomach,' he says, 'is fear and panic.' For this reason, Simeons classified those infectious diseases which enter the body *via* the stomach (bacillary dysentery and typhoid as well as cholera) as partially psychosomatic illnesses, since mental factors help to elect the epidemic victims. Simeons was at pains to exclude insect-borne diseases such as bubonic plague, malaria and yellow fever, and his theory does not even explain the continued good health of Pettenkofer, since the cholera bug *did* reach his intestine. However, Simeons was writing in 1960, since when there has been an explosion of research into the immune system. It is here that we must seek explanations for Pettenkofer's happy result, and for evidence in favour of Dr Johnson's dictum.

The immune system

I have already described two great channels of communication in the body, the nervous and the hormonal systems. It has only become clear in this century that there is another system sending messages around the body which is just as vital to life and survival. A significant part of this system has already been described: the hormonal memoranda sent by the body to adjust the operations of such organs as the kidneys, alimentary tract and sex organs. But hormones are not the end of the story. In addition to the chemical memoranda, the body's homeostatic bureacracy has a number of active service units in the field.

We owe the notion of a *milieu intérieure* to Pasteur's distinguished rival, Claude Bernard, and today Bernard would

106

undoubtedly have referred to an *ecology* of the body – a concept very different from the image of 'man-the-machine' which had gained such wide popularity in the eighteenth and early nineteenth centuries. Bernard's innovation was to see the body as a controlled habitat for living cells whose most urgent biological needs are to co-operate successfully with 'friends' and to combat 'enemies' – enemies being defined as alien or not–Self and friends as Self, with a few useful microbial squatters who are treated as honorary parts of Self. These latter are beneficial parasites, keeping down other bacteria and, in some cases, helping to synthesize useful vitamins – a highly homeostatic relationship between host and parasite known as 'symbiosis'. Other bacteria, on the other hand, are potentially harmful and it is these which must be dealt with by the mobilization of our own defences, the vital biological task carried out largely by the cells of the immune system – the white-blood cells, or leucocytes – with assistance from such chemical agents as the interferons.

In spite of Bernard's ecological milieu, the immune system seems irresistibly like a parody of certain theories of police work. Some of its defensive cells, the phagocytes, constitute an elite squad. Their detail is to patrol the bloodstream, taking alien bacteria into custody and liquidating them. At points of damage, they leave the bloodstream and crowd together in the tissue, helped there by the release of histamine which dilates blood vessels and thins their walls. This allows fluids to pass into damaged tissue from the blood vessels: hence the swelling that follows some infections and injuries, and hence ultimately the pus, made of the burnt-out phagocytes which are the end-products of the process. There is, however, another division of the leucocytes, cells produced in the lymph glands called lymphocytes; these are of even greater significance, since it is through them that the all-important antibodies are deployed.

It is startling to realize the sheer number of living foreign bodies – most of them micro-organisms – which settle inside the body as a result of breathing, feeding and injury. Bacteria, the germs with which Pasteur made his name, vary in size but all seem incredibly small at first acquaintance since thousands can crowd on to the surface of the tiniest visible speck of dust. Their other quality is speed of reproduction, so quick that in fabourable conditions there will be a million where ten hours earlier there was only one.

Bacteria are an indeterminate entity somewhere between animal and vegetable, thus they can be attacked by chemicals (antibiotics) which destroy the enzymes they need for metabolism. Not so the viruses; these are graded in size between the smallest bacteria and the largest chemical molecules, but on average are a thousand times smaller than bacteria. Viruses would be the tiniest living things on earth if we could be really sure that they are alive. Sometimes they behave as if they were (they reproduce), yet they are utterly incapable of independent activity being too small to contain the necessary metabolic material. It follows that, having no enzymes, they cannot be killed by enzyme-destroying chemicals and also that, to achieve their destiny, viruses must latch on to living cells whose metabolizing chemistry (the cell's enzymes) they can take over for their own ends.

Although it has only a tiny amount of nucleic acid (DNA, or in some cases RNA), there is enough to go to work on the cell's own RNA which is the chemical constituent of its genes. The virus disconnects the cell's genes and plugs in the genetic programme contained in its own DNA/RNA. The cell is then entirely disabled and at the disposal of the virus, which proceeds to replicate itself as fast as it can until the cell bursts and the vast brood of newborn viruses is unleashed on neighbouring cells. If this happens on a large scale, the host organism itself will be in great danger and the host's security forces must again be called out.

In theory, these defences are good enough eventually to extinguish any threat. Phagocytes are useless against free viruses, but the lymphocyte division of the immune system is specially designed to shackle them. If an unfamiliar antigen (i.e. a not-Self protein) is discovered in the body, some obscure 'research' facility in the immune system begins work on the design of an antibody – a cell which is chemically complementary to the *particular* antigen detected, and which 'fits' the antigen as precisely as a key fits a lock. Within a week or so, the antibody is perfected and the lymphocyte cells then go into full wartime production. Once released in the body, the antibodies seek out and handcuff the antigens, which can then only await their fate at the hands of the phagocytes. Once a particular antigen has been faced and dealt with in this way, a few copies of its appropriate antibody are retained, to be used as templates in case they are needed again. This is immunity, exactly the same as the state conferred by innoculation. It means that there is no delay in the production of antibodies a second, third or fourth time around, so that in immune people the disease is aborted before any symptoms appear.

So it is normally the first attack of a virus that causes the worst mischief, if any. The polio virus, for example, gets into the grey matter in the front part of the spinal cord, where nerve cells control the contraction of muscles. Extensive viral damage to spinal nerve cells may be caused before sufficient antibodies have been produced to prevent it. Unfortunately this damage is permanent, because unlike most other cells, nerve cells cannot regenerate, hence the paralysis which affects serious cases. But polio victims who survive cannot contract the disease again.

Thus it can be seen that the immune system entails highly sophisticated biological processes involving, for instance, pattern-recognition and memory, two skills which are basic to mind itself. Does this mean, though, that the mind is in any way a participant in the system? For instance, does the unshakable confidence of a von Pettenkoffer confer an immunity which on purely mechanistic grounds he should not enjoy? Or is immunity a separate and automatic physiological department, a 'closed system' answerable only to itself? Of course, a holistic approach does not on principle accept that bodily systems can be completely closed. But, as Dr Samuel Johnson would have been interested to know, even rational objective scientific analysis is now beginning to bear out his thesis, 190 years after his death.

Mind and immunity

Everybody knows that nobody knows the cure for the common cold. There are many mysteries about colds, but most boil down to the more general mystery of our unpredictable response to all viral challenges. For instance, we become *infected* with colds, on average, once a month. But, again on average, we actually develop a cold only three of four times a year.

At the Common Cold Research Unit in Salisbury, Wiltshire, volunteers are willing to place themselves in the hands of scientists and take the chance of catching a stinker of a cold in return for ten days' free holiday. It is an ideal population of human laboratory specimens for studying how and why people become infected with a virus and how and why only some of those infected go on to develop symptoms.

For example, psychologists carried out personality tests on these volunteers in 1980 and 1985 and identified certain individuals who were more likely to catch colds in any given trial. Introverted people were relatively more likely to succumb, as were those who had recently experienced major changes in their lives such as a new job, marriage, a fortieth birthday, divorce, retirement or bereavement.

Why? A common genetic cause may be a possible explanation of the link between introversion and susceptibility to colds, but this could not explain the influence of life changes since they are (or can be) random. The effects of stress and the response to it, varying from one individual to another, seem much more plausible and promising areas of investigation.

The American scientist Michael Plaut has done intensive research into the immune systems of mice under stress. The first stressor he looked at was overcrowding. He infected mice with a malarial parasite whose effect is specific to rodents and found that their survival was strongly influenced by the number of mice in the cage; overcrowded mice produced fewer antibodies and died sooner. Plaut also looked at the stresses caused by aggression and fear. Resistance to a tapeworm parasite was significantly but temporarily lowered both in mice who had been fighting and mice who were shown to a cat.[7]

However, this is very complex and variable. Different species do not show uniform suppression of immunity under stress, nor do varieties of the same species as might be expected. The effect also varies according to the strain of the virus present and the type of stress. Testing mouse immunity against one pathogen known as virus Coxsackie B, Plaut tried the effects of exposing them to bright lights and random electric shocks. He found that both stressors combined significantly lowered antibody production, while the electric shocks alone had no effect. With a completely different virus, however – the mouse-malaria virus – both shock-and-light and shock alone lowered immune response by the same amount. So extrapolation from one species (mice) to another (men) is clearly hazardous.

Another of Plaut's findings was that, if he *isolated* a mouse in a cage away from its fellows, immunity was significantly damaged, apparently as a direct effect of loneliness. The question for human medicine then is: can effects like these be observed in people? How much correspondence is there between the immune responses of mice and men?

In humans a useful virus in studying this is *herpes simplex*, responsible for cold sores. Following a first infection, it lies doggo in the body until immunity is again low enough to reawaken it. Over the past five years, researchers at Ohio State University have found that there is more herpes activity and less immune reactivity among medical students stressed by examinations than in those not stressed. However, when these students feld *lonely*, their immune systems worked even more lamely.[8] Work published in 1984 by Stephen Schliefer and colleagues at Mount Sinai in New York showed that two months after bereavement a group of widowers had depressed immunity, as compared with measurements taken just before their wives died. Looking at separation and divorce – which for some time have been known to increase short-term mortality from pneumonia and TB in both sexes – the team from Ohio State have found herpes to be more active in women recently separated and divorced. According to their measurements, the more these women had loved their husbands the greater the immunity deficit when the separation occurred.

The immune system has its own memory: it never forgets a face. The memory of those first exposures to smallpox, chicken-pox, measles and mumps is what confers lifelong immunity. Vaccination, then, is nothing but the *education* of the leucocytes in pathogen-recognition. Work by Robert Ader and Nicholas Cohen of the University of Rochester, New York, shows that immunity is also hooked up to our mental memory circuits, and that these too can activate or suppress it.

Ader and Cohen did this by making use of Pavlovian conditioning. The Russian neurologist Ivan Pavlov (1849–1936) investigated the reflex mechanism whereby a hungry dog salivates copiously at the sight of food – what he called an unconditioned (i.e. natural) reflex. He and his team found that, if for a certain period they always associated the arrival of food with the ringing of a bell, the dog's saliva glands could eventually be induced to work at the sound of the bell *alone*. This was the famous *conditioned* or artificial reflex; it showed how the brain and nervous system processed the body's automatic procedures centrally, which were thereby proved to be not merely the result of local stimuli.

Ader and Cohen wondered whether immunity itself could be conditioned. They put a number of laboratory rats on regular injections of cyclophosphamide, a drug which automatically depresses the immune system. This was their unconditioned immunosuppressive reflex. They then produced an artificial association with this reflex by always giving the injection at the same time as a drink of saccharine-flavoured water. After a time, the rats showed exactly the same depressed immunity if given a drink of saccharine water alone, as had been caused by cyclophosphamide.

So the immune system looks as if it is susceptible to conditioning, but conditioning itself is a deterministic principle which does not admit the possibility of choice. Hence, since I have laid much stress on the idea that choice plays a part in psychosomatic events, the role of conditioning should perhaps be examined in a little more detail.

Conditioning

Pavlov's initial interest was in showing the brain's involvement in automatic processes like the production of saliva and gastric juices. For instance, he proved that if you put food directly into the stomach without it being *eaten* it cannot be digested. The act of digestion is triggered by the act of tasting and eating, *via* the brain – a circuit which in part we have already seen working in reverse, when the flow of stomach acids is blocked by anxiety during a cholera epidemic. However, Pavlov proceeded to develop a generalized psychology which saw unconditioned reflexes as not merely the basis of the autonomic nervous system, but of all instinctive *behaviour*. He went on to assert that deliberate behaviour – in animals certainly, and in man to a very great extent – could be regarded as little more than a highly complex pattern of *conditioned* reflexes. Conditioning then became another way of talking about the process of learning.

But if that is *all* there is to learning – the accumulation of 'correct' reflexes – our freedom and our humanity evaporate.

Far from enjoying free will, in this unappealing psychology we are prisoners of the Pavlovian response, either conditioned or otherwise. Such thinking is one of the foundation planks of modern behaviourism, which in its extreme form we have seen to be utterly inimical to the whole notion of psychosomatic disease. B. F. Skinner, the foremost living behaviourist, denies the existence of any such disease.

But even if we disagree with mechanical behaviourism, we cannot gainsay conditioning: it exists and is in fact a crucially important part of our mental lives, often agonizingly so. Much of our behaviour is conditioned by experiences and associations over which we have little or no control, especially early experiences. Of all physiological processes, none is more easily and variously conditioned than the sexual response. The wealth of emotional and spiritual consequences from this fact alone is practically inexhaustible; we have seen examples of the darker side of it in Rousseau and T. E. Lawrence, but what do we make of a case quoted by Havelock Ellis – that of a doctor 'of unimpeachable morality who was unable to attend funerals, even of his own relatives, on account of the sexual excitement thus aroused'?[9]

Eating is another typically susceptible activity. In China they breed Chow dogs for the table; in the Middle East a sheep's eye is the delicacy reserved for the most favoured guest; and in South-East Asia journalist Estelle Holt 'watched a group of Lao peasants watching a USAID agricultural adviser milk a cow and then drink the milk. They were intrigued and revolted, and when offered a glass of the stuff, even their natural courtesy could hardly conceal disgust'.[10] In earliest times the inhabitants of a cave at Choukoutien, near Peking, are thought to have eaten the brains of their deceased relatives before burial. Americans and Europeans would certainly gag and retch uncontrollably if forced to swallow such a meal. The primitive Choukoutienese would surely have done likewise at mouthfuls of Mars bar, or cheese and onion crisps.

Conditioning does still more; it affects the entire imaginative quality of life and of memory. Tiny inconspicuous events can have far-reaching consequences for the personality, something which has never been more memorably exploited than by Marcel Proust. In his great work of a million and a quarter words, the little episode of the madeleine cake assumes gigantic importance. This is one of the most frequently cited passages in modern literature but, like the rest of the novel, it is rarely read. The narrator accidentally drops a piece of the cake into his tea, retrieves it with a spoon and tastes it. At once he is suffused by extraordinary pleasure, a sense of inner transfiguration which at first he cannot explain. With effort, however, he does at last dredge up a memory from his childhood: those apparently inconsequential Sunday mornings when his Aunt Leonie, sitting up in bed, let him eat a morsel of her breakfast madeleine after first dipping it in her cup of tea. It was a completely private and subjective experience, not one whose power Ivan Pavlov or B. F. Skinner would recognize, yet upon it the whole *Remembrance of Things Past* pivots. This unexploded bomb had lain dormant throughout the intervening years:

> . . . but when from a long-distant past nothing subsists, after the people are dead, after the things are broken or scattered, taste and smell alone, more fragile but more enduring, more unsubstantial, more persistent, more faithful, remain poised a long time, like souls, remembering, waiting, hoping, amid the ruins of all the rest; and bear unflinchingly, in the tiny and almost impalpable drop of their essence, the vast structure of recollection.[11]

The complex of tastes and smells surrounding these childhood moments had become embedded in Proust's mind. Then, like a charge blowing off the door of a safe, the re-enacted combination of cake and tea exploded in the adult Proust's mind with overwhelming force. This can only be attributed to a kind of conditioning.

So conditioning can enfold a key to vast storehouses of human memory and remembered sensation, but that does not imply that it is the only key, or that it is a limiting and imprisoning key: for Proust, the madeleine was not confining but liberating. Freud makes the same point. Psychoanalysis is nothing if it does not reach back and turn those keys of memory which reveal the unconscious mind. Conditioning, then, is one way in which memory links are forged, in which parts of ourselves are formed. But when it comes to explaining the whole of consciousness, individuality, personality, emotion and above all reason, the Pavlovian discoveries are only a beginning.

It seems that the more random a piece of early conditioning

is, the more powerfully it can rebound later in life, the more trouble it causes. The respectable doctor unable to attend funerals and the war hero with an obsessive urge to be flogged are tragic victims of cruel but chance associations, probably experienced in childhood, which at the time were of little observable importance. For whatever complex of psychological reasons, these trivialities nevertheless took root in their imaginations. Once welded into place there, they formed disturbing and inappropriate stimulus-response circuits, which in turn led to impulses causing daily agony and shame in the adult who still carried them with him.

The body also forms inappropriate stimulus-response circuits which are usually established in early childhood – the muscular tics and other involuntary writhings of Dr Johnson, for example. More internal to the body, and dealing not with the psychological but the immune memory, we have the phenomenon of *allergy*.

Allergy

Every year there is a pandemic which affects three million people in Britain and hundreds of millions in Europe and North America. Initially, the eyes and nose itch and there is a feeling of tension behind the upper face. A profuse watery discharge from the eyes and nose follows, as does a headache and violent sneezing. Perhaps 15 per cent of sufferers feel extremely ill and are unable to function properly. We call the disease hay fever, though there is usually no rise in temperature.

Treatment consists simply of staying away from grass – the source of the pollen which causes the malady. Hay fever has a sister syndrome, a rhinitis which is not seasonal and whose cause is very much more difficult to avoid. This is the harmless house-dust mite, a minute creature which infests the domestic environment, especially beds, cushions, and upholstery or wherever it finds the greatest concentration of its favourite food – cast-off human skin cells. Wherever dust is disturbed, the mite is breathed in.

Most symptoms of illness are a perfectly correct response to an environmental threat. Coughing brings up sputum and is one way of expelling unwanted germs from the body; shivering warms; skin pallor is a sign that blood supply has been diverted to essential organs. It is even now suspected that fever – for long regarded as an unfortunate side-effect of illness or infection – may have the useful function of helping to cook microbes to death. But with allergy the symptoms arise quite simply from a mistake. The body's immune system trips into action at the presence of a harmless or inert protein and treats this allergen like an antigen – a poison or a deadly micro-organism. This happens when the immune system is conditioned or 'sensitized' during an initial exposure to the protein, and thereafter, whenever this allergen is encountered the symptoms appear. Nobody knows why this piece of conditioning happens when it does.

So, with allergy, the symptoms of infection or injury are simulated. Antibodies are produced which combine with the allergens detected in the body and this leads to the release of histamine and other chemicals. Sometimes even more dramatic changes occur, most often during allergic responses to infrequent – but still relatively harmless – stimuli such as bee-stings. This is the infamous *anaphylactic shock* which results in coma and, unless treated, in death.

It is the histamine and other released chemicals (leukotrines and prostaglandins) that cause most of the physical signs of an allergic response. These chemicals are essential components of the immune system and their normal function is to assist leucocytes to concentrate within threatened or damaged tissue. They dilate the blood vessels in the area of perceived danger and swelling occurs – normally beneficial, though in allergy this may become the unsightly skin condition of urticaria. Further side-effects of these chemicals are a headache and perhaps a blocked nose. Their release can also cause the constriction of the bronchial muscles which provokes the respiratory distress in asthma, and the secretions from the eyes, nose and ears typical of hay fever. We need to remember that, where the immune system is dealing with an *antigen*, these effects are necessary and even life-saving; but where the foe is a harmless *allergen* they are nothing but *side*-effects, an unnecessary discomfort.

Unnecessary? That would seem so. Yet the association between immune response and the mind is so secure – and at least in allergy's case is now fairly respectable with doctors –

that it becomes necessary to ask whether the allergy has some subjective meaning, some private *necessity*.

MESSAGE FROM A CORK-LINED ROOM

Marcel Proust's hypersensitive nature was governed according to a turning wheel of health and ill-health. From the age of nine he had been attacked by disabling bouts of asthma and hay fever, which at the start coincided with the summer pollen season. Gradually through his teens, the attacks became worse though their association with the pollen count grew less important. He himself came to realize that the rhythm of his attacks was now more to do with the emotional climate, in particular with the rise and fall of his feelings about his mother and of hers about him.

Proust and his mother enjoyed a quite exceptional interdependence – a cloying, clinging love which strait-laced Professor Proust, Marcel's doctor father, found quite distasteful. When he still lived with his parents, there were nights when Proust's asthma prevented him from sleeping. He would then write long letters to his Mamma, leaving them in the hall for her to read while he slept all day. In one of these, written when he was twenty-seven, he seemed to realize that their relationship had scarcely matured since the date of his first attack eighteen years before. Since that time his happiness had been utterly bound up with hers and hers with his illness, for this represented the continuance of her son's dependence on her maternal tenderness. So, in a way, he saw it as part of his filial duty to continue to be sickly. In one of his letters he wrote:

'The truth is that when I feel well, the sort of life that keeps me exasperates you to the point of demolishing it, until I fall ill again. . . . It really is miserable not to be able to to enjoy health and affection simultaneously'.[12]

And in another:

'I would so much rather please you, even if it meant having an attack, than displease you and be spared one . . .'[13]

Proust was always hypersensitive to noise. After his mother's death, when writing *Remembrance of Things Past*, he had a room in his flat at 102 Boulevard Haussmann entirely cork-lined, ostensibly to exclude the sound of nearby building works. However, this famous piece of insulation has assumed symbolic

117

importance for Proust's biographers, emphasizing the sick man's own insulation from the world of health and of the present tense. This insulation was in fact essential in order for the creative artist in Proust to be released, since his project was to recreate the past; so by cultivating his own weakness he nurtured the strength of his book. By the end of his life (and towards the end of writing the book) he became an entirely nocturnal creature, sleeping by day only with the help of veronal, living like some alchemist in a dense cloud of breath-assisting fumigatory smoke. He saw hardly anybody, ate rarely and then would take only food brought from restaurants, since the faintest smell of cooking in the house provoked violent asthma. In these ways did his disease, which had once served his mother, now serve his art.

What on earth would Proust have done if anti-histamine inhalers had been invented? Anti-histamines, which first appeared from the Pasteur Institute in 1937, have revolutionized the lives of modern asthmatics.

Proust would still have had plenty of alternative pathologies to choose from. We have covered the skin diseases and all the varieties of pain syndrome which might have been available to him, but there are also a number of bowel disorders to hand – dangerous ones such as Crohn's disease and ulcerative colitis, and more 'benign' conditions like diverticulitis and spastic colon, not to mention a goodly range of inflammatory conditions including rheumatoid arthritis and migraine.

This last example is a little understood malady. It recurs with an almost tidal frequency, though there is a possible connection with the immune system. As neurologist Oliver Sacks argues, migraine often strongly suggests an element of unconscious motivation. Two case histories from his book *Migraine* show this with exceptional clarity.

OPTIONAL ALLERGY

A twenty-four-year-old patient of Dr Sacks had suffered from serious asthma between the ages of eight and thirteen. From his teens, however, the asthma disappeared to be replaced by a regular Sunday afternoon migraine. Sacks's treatment, probably with ergotamine drugs, was able to abolish all symptoms, but instead of being grateful this patient returned angrily to the consulting room a few weeks later demanding his migraines back. It turned out that in between times his old asthma had returned, worse than he had originally known it, and he found this much more inconvenient than the weekly migraines.[14]

Another patient of this remarkable neurologist kept three conditions running in endless circular relay – a case far more tragic and disturbing than that of Proust, who at least had the consolation of genius and creative release. This woman, too, had made her existential choice, which led her under a darker shadow of suffering than those who knew her can ever have realized. I describe her in Sack's own words:

> A fifty-five-year-old woman, unmarried, and the only daughter of parents who had always been demanding and possessive, and who were now ageing and in poor health, she was compelled to work at two jobs, for a total of fourteen hours daily, to support the household. She had no friends, no social life, and had never had any sexual experience. She felt it her duty to support her parents and to be with them when she was not working.
>
> At one time she had made pathetic efforts to establish an independent existence, but these had been foiled at first by parental intervention, and subsequently by her own discomfort and guilt if she went out alone. In the past ten years she had lost all choice in the matter, for she suffered severely from migraine, ulcerative colitis and psoriasis, not concurrently, but in a never-ending cycle.[15]

In conclusion, we might ask where such choices are made: where the mind and the body's chemical communication system interact; where, perhaps, von Pettenkofer was saved from cholera; and from where we can trace the path which drew Proust into his cork-lined room. We might ask, but it would be over-optimistic to expect an answer. There is no single *location* in the brain for existential decision-making. The hypothalamus is important, because it regulates the thymus gland where t-cells are made and has other responsibilities in the immune system. But immunity is a system which operates like a network. It carries out functions such as the detection of foreign material in the body, but at a higher level of organization it also helps the organism to define itself.

So the discovery and investigation of the immune system has

revealed much about the way in which complex systems of organization in the body – neural and biochemical ones, for instance – combine and interpenetrate to keep the organism itself in existence. It has also brought the germ theory itself into perspective. Germs are not like rats trying to escape from a sack, gnawing holes in the fabric and more or less incidentally ruining the sack. The ruin, if it occurs, is done with the sack's own help and connivance.

Pasteur is supposed to have put it another way on his deathbed. 'Bernard was right,' he is reported to have muttered. 'The microbe is nothing, the terrain everything!'

Chapter 6

Self against self

'Nothing could be more vivid than
their language,
Lethal, sparkling and irregular stars,
The murderous design of the universe,
The hectic dance of the passionate
cancer cells.'
The Cancer Cells – Richard Eberhardt

*T*he lines are from a poem in which Eberhardt describes the beauty he sees in some photographs of cancer cells taken through a microscope. His enthusiasm looks like a deliberate provocation. He claims an artistic fellow-feeling with the cells, with their anarchic destructiveness, their blind cosmic purposes and their 'quick and lean' design. Pehaps most significantly of all, he sees 'my own malignance in their racy, beautiful gestures'. For most people, these are precisely the features of cancer which terrify.

It sometimes seems that cancer has come into its inheritance in our times. We are less in peril of death under the age of forty than at any period in history, which means that we place more time at the disposal of latent cancers. But also we live *differently* now: we are more stressed, polluted and irradiated; less religious and rooted; more lonely, desperate, paranoid, drug-addicted, emotionally disturbed, hurried, urbanized. In short, we are more *civilized*.

Under these conditions cancer has flourished and now accounts for almost a quarter of UK deaths, which is an increase of 180 per cent on the cancer death-rate of 1911–15.[1] The breast cancer death-rate has more than doubled in this century. Pancreatic cancer, a rare disease before the First World War, has increased more than five-fold, and the death rate from lung cancers (35,739 in 1984) is still increasing. Leukaemias and lympahatic cancers (8,687 deaths in 1984) have increased since 1915 by the greatest factor of all – six or seven times, which is only partially explicable in terms of improvements in diagnosis. Prostate cancer, to which older men are particularly vulnerable, claims seven times more victims (6,248 in 1984) than seventy years ago, and is also increasing year by year.

Fig. 3. Cancer Survival: percentage surviving five years or more after diagnosis of 10 common cancers in England and Wales

Site of Cancer	Women					Men				
	1947	1958	1966	1975	1982	1947	1958	1966	1975	1982
Pancreas	n/a	2	2	3·6	2·6	n/a	2	2	2·8	2·6
Lung	3	4	5	6·6	6·3	2	6	6	7	5·9
Stomach	n/a	5	6	7·4	7·4	n/a	7	6	6·9	7
Colon	18	25	27	29·5	26·8	15	23	25	31·3	26·5
Rectum	22	27	30	30·6	27·9	17	26	29	30·6	27
Ovary	n/a	21	24	23·4	26·8	–	–	–	–	–
Prostate	–	–	–	–	–	24	27	32	35·1	29·7
Breast	37	44	53	57·4	55·1	–	–	–	–	–
Cervix	35	43	67	51·7	51·8	–	–	–	–	–
Skin	77	84	81	97·4	78·4	78	86	80	96·4	83·7

Source: Office of Population and Censuses.

In response to these alarming figures, amounting in the case of lung, breast and some other cancers to an epidemic, the warning bells started ringing in the period after the Second World War. Today, forty years of intensive medical research later, the situation has improved for some varieties of the disease, notably skin cancers, leukaemia and cancers in children generally. The death-rate from cancer for patients under the age of fourteen, for example, has fallen by 25 per cent in twenty years. However, for the more common cancers results have been very much less encouraging. There has been an increase in the number of women with breast cancer who survive five years after diagnosis (37 per cent in 1947 as against 57.4 per cent thirty years later), but this is thought to have been partly the result of earlier detection. For most cancers, there is little clear evidence that screening programmes, early dectection and variations in treatment make very much difference to life-expectancy. Carcinoma of the lung (from which most patients die within two years) has remained almost universally untreatable, as we can see by comparing the reported lung cancer incidence in one year with its mortality in the next. In 1983, 35,922 cases of malignancy in the lung, trachea and bronchus were reported in England and Wales. In 1984, the recorded death-rate from these diseases was 35,739. No wonder this is the most feared illness of the northern, Westernised, post-Christian world.

Fear in itself can cause death. It can certainly lower resistance and initiate disease. Therefore the fear inspired by cancer presents us with a circle from which it is hard to break free: the disease spurring us on to spur on the disease. This closed wheel encapsulates the secrets of cancer's peculiar power. However, there is a second circle of tautology lying within the first.

If we ask, 'Where does the fear of cancer come from? Is it inherently any more frightful than other diseases?' We must, I think, answer with a qualified 'Yes'. At this stage of our species' development cancer *is* inherently frightful; we can hardly avoid perceiving it so, with the effect of making ourselves fear it all the more. That is the second circle: fear engendering more of the same. The reason for cancer's fundamental horror is found in the way it is generated out of our own cells.

The cancer cells make us afraid because in their glassy malevolence we cannot help recognizing – as Eberhardt does – our own image, our own progeny. They are like children who have deliberately set out to extirpate their own families. Familial quarrels and rebellion are the stuff of Greek tragedy – man's first really sophisticated artistic response to experience – and are major themes in a good half of Shakespeare's plays. The kinds of emotion which such themes evoke, from embarrassment and lurking discomfort to full-blown terror, are perfectly mirrored in our feelings about cancer.

This is the clue to Richard Eberhardt's paradoxical delight in the cancer cells. The poet recognizes in them a purity and passion for destruction which he cannot help admiring: aesthetic fascism, though unattractive, is by no means rare in literature. It is also a clear starting point for the exploration of cancer as a psychosomatic illness, a 'disease which speaks'.

Our first problem is of identity. Just what are these cancer cells? Are they foreign tissue or part of the Self? Subjectively this can be cleared up quickly enough, because even though we might try to imagine otherwise (as Eberhardt does) we cannot really feel that cancer is a Martian invader, landing secretly on the planets of our stomach, breasts or lungs entirely from its own expansionist motives.

If the image of invaders is rejected, would we do better to see the cells of a tumour as parasites? A parasite lodges in our bodies because they are warm and nutritious, though it is as happy to doss down anywhere else given an equally agreeable ambience. The trouble with this idea is that it is fundamentally against the interests of a parasite to destroy the host. A parasite's evolutionary purpose (if 'purpose' is allowable) is to live in symbiosis with the host – to be left alone to live, like the beat poet Lawrence Ferlinghetti in his *Autobiography*, 'a quiet life in Mike's place':

> watching the world walk by
> in its curious shoes.

Certainly some parasites – infective bacteria, for example – do not achieve this. Their presence in the body causes irritation and threatens disease, or even death. Knowing this, the immune system then moves into action against them. In the same way, Ferlinghetti's host Mike might finally become exasperated with the laconic idle poet and throw him into the street. However, there is a time-lag (for the pathogen, if not the poet) before nemesis strikes. The bacteria not only reproduces very fast and so can complete many thousands of life-cycles in a few hours, it can also move rapidly between hosts, enabling the species to keep one step ahead of the game. Cancer is different. The effect of cancer cell reproduction is not because it is too fast – it need take only thirty divisions to produce a pea-sized tumour containing a billion cells – but because it is *uncontrolled*.

An even more fundamental difference is that our parasites are in no sense a part of us, any more than Ferlinghetti is part of Mike. If they were, they could not be parasites. By contrast, our cancer cells are rather ambivalent in their relationship with us. They show some characteristics in common with the otherness of parasites (and with the alien-ness of Martian invaders), yet we are quite sure that they are by and large spontaneously generated from within. To understand this more clearly we shall need to embark upon a fairly lengthy diversion through the twisted history of DNA.

Carcinogenesis

Nestling in the nucleus of every cell are the double-spirals of deoxyribonucleic acid, or DNA. These are the beginning of life and the necessary condition of its continuation. Without the step-by-step instructions which these molecules carry, a cell simply does not exist: it cannot even make the proteins needed to maintain its own shape, let alone to carry out functions within the organism. DNA, then, is a detailed cell-by-cell specification for the organism, unique to each individual and written in a genetic code which uses a chemical alphabet.

A simplified sketch of the architecture of this system would have to start with the packets of DNA joining together to form units of heredity, generally called genes. The genes in turn are strung together, like unclasped necklaces (between 20,000 and 90,000 genes to each string), to form chromosomes. These chromosomes hold hands in pairs. There are twenty-three pairs of them in each and every cell of the human body with the sole exception of the 'half-cells' of reproduction, the sperm and the ova. These half-cells have twenty-three unpaired chromosomes and can become complete only by fertilization.

Apart from the reproductive purpose of the gametes, all cells naturally need to reproduce themselves if tissue is to grow or regrow, and this is done by splitting. It is this process of cell splitting which in cancer is out of control, but it is also at the crucial moment when a normal cell splits that the initial cancer cell is born. So what happens when a cell splits?

The pairs of spiralling strings of DNA, holding on to each other like dancing partners, are made up from only four molecules: thymine, cytosine, guanine and adenine. These four molecules (called 'bases') are the symbols or letters used by the genetic language, as dots and dashes are those employed by morse. So it is the order of the four bases along the DNA strings which constitutes the detailed biological specification.

Before a cell divides the spiral pairs separate, as if unplugged, and dance away into opposite halves of the cell. A new cell wall forms between them, so now two cells exist where before there was one. The separated spirals of DNA within the new cells are only without a partner for a very short time. Each base along the string sets about reconstructing its opposite number and in this way all the double spirals are re-made and reiterated in each new cell and in all succeeding generations of cell.

However the system is not perfect, and 'misprints' in the specification occur. Where such misprints happen in the gamete, the result may be the birth of a new mutant individual whose characteristics are passed on to succeeding generations and perhaps retained in the species. If, on the other hand, the mutation occurs during splitting in any of the other non-reproductive cells, the normal result is that the next generation of cell fails to survive; it becomes simply a manufacturing reject. However, in some cases the mutation may preserve or even reinforce a particular cell's integrity. If that cell's ability to divide is also preserved, it will survive and reproduce itself, perhaps giving rise to a tumour. If, in addition, it somehow knows how to evade or disconnect the homeostatic mechanisms which normally turn cell division on and off, a swift uncontrolled and aggressive new growth – 'neoplasm' – begins to flourish. This is the malignancy of cancer.

An alternative genetic explanation of carcinogenesis is that for some reason the genes for uncontrolled growth ('oncogenes') already exist, so that some – or all – of us are pre-programmed as potential cancer victims. On this theory, these genes are equipped with a safety catch which stays firmly in the 'off' position unless and until something happens to throw them across to 'on'.

The unifying characteristics of all cancer cells, then, are that they result either from a misprint in their genetic message or from the unleashing of a previously restrained oncogene, and that they behave in the same way – reproducing aggressively, selfishly and incontinently without regard for the welfare of the neighbouring tissue. They are the delinquent prodigal children of law-abiding cells. But what causes the mutation, or throws the oncogene switch?

Carcinogens

A carcinogen is any influence which provokes the growth of neoplasms. Many of these are quite well-known: radiation, toxic chemicals and viruses. They all irritate the cell and, depending upon which theory you prefer, either switch on the oncogene or cause the mutation which sets the cancer cell going. Either way, they presumably do this by *shock* or *sustained irritation* of the cells concerned. The first known chemical carcinogen was soot, recognized by the London surgeon Percival Pott in 1775. He noticed that the unlucky chimney-sweeps, who in those days cleaned flues by climbing down them, suffered commonly from cancer of the scrotum. Later, coal tar was identified as carcinogenic when nineteenth-century dye workers producing coal-tar dyes were found to have a high incidence of skin and bladder cancer. Arsenic and asbestos are also carcinogenic and so, most famously of all, is cigarette smoke.

X-rays and other forms of radiation were discovered to be carcinogenic the hard way. It has been estimated that from 1902 onwards, at least a hundred early X-ray workers died from the disease. Both Marie Curie and her daughter died from leukaemia. We are now very much more careful in the use of X-rays, but this attitude is of quite recent origin. Many people will remember as children up to the 1950s being allowed to *play* with the foot X-ray machines which used to be a vaunted feature of all the plusher shoe-shops.

However, none of these influences causes cancer by simple or occasional contamination. They have their effect over long periods, even years, of daily exposure. Nevertheless, children are apparently much more susceptible to some environmental carcinogens, as was shown when a higher rate of leukaemia was found in children living near the nuclear reprocessing plant at Sellafield in Cumbria.

With their direct effect on the nucleic acid of cells, viruses at one time looked to be promising subjects for cancer research. Animals exposed to certain viruses do develop a number of cancers. If suckled by a mouse from a cancer-prone strain, baby mice of a cancer-resistant strain usually get cancer, from a virus originally called 'the milk factor'. But early hopes that viruses are a common cause of all cancers have been dashed, though a few are convincingly linked with particular cancers. The Epstein-Barr Virus is associated with Burkitt's Lymphoma, a disease largely of African children. The human T-cell leukaemia virus (HTLV-1) was identified in the late seventies, and more recent evidence has linked a wart-causing virus (human papillomavirus) with cancers of the skin and especially the cervix. Herpes, too – like HTLV-1, a retrovirus which lies low in the body for years – may be carcinogenic in some people. Even better known today is the AIDS virus. AIDS victims usually develop an otherwise rare skin cancer called Kaposi's sarcoma, but this is regarded as a consequence of the virus's primary damage – the destruction of the healthy immune response.

These are all environmental carcinogenic influences which can sometimes cause trauma inside the cell and nudge the oncogene switch, or – by causing damage – trigger a mutation in the normal DNA. But like so much else in cancer research, the quest for specific sure-fire environmental carcinogens – though at various times it has seemed promising – has ultimately proved a fool's errand. Even factors which are demonstrably carcinogenic do not have an inevitable effect. Nine out of ten heavy cigarette smokers never get lung cancer, nor do most asbestos workers. The terrible legacy of the Hiroshima and Nagasaki disasters has included a greatly increased rate of death from cancer amongst survivors, especially leukaemia and thyroid cancer. Yet the length of time before these appeared (if they have done so) has been extremely variable and uncertain. Ronald Bodley Scott, a British authority on cancer, underlines this point in his book *Cancer: The Facts*:

In patients with leukaemia, the frequency with which a story of exposure to ionizing radiation can be obtained is not above 3 or 4 per cent. Similarly the cancer of the liver which workers in the polyvinyl chloride industry may develop is one of exceptional rarity. *In the vast majority of patients the cancer arises spontaneously and none of the causal factors discussed can be inculpated.*[2]

There are of course millions of influences at work in the *internal* environment of the body. We have seen the orchestration of the hormones by those parts of the brain which also process our emotions. Other body chemicals such as neurotransmitters and enzymes, with the immune system itself, are equally active and equally affected by the mind. So, given our failure to find *external* carcinogens which can unfailingly cause human cancer, the next logical place to look is inside ourselves – in the body and, inevitably therefore, in the mind.

The nature of cancer

So we come back to that intangible *personal* quality of this disease. Bodley Scott writes about cancer's nature that: 'it is impossible to define it more exactly than to say that the disorder is one of uncontrolled and purposeless growth – indeed, no single other feature has been identified as common to all cancer cells and it is possible that none exists'.[3] If cancer is indeed linked to the personality, this might seem less baffling; though far from simplifying the scientific problem, it must make it more difficult. Personalities differ from each other much too radically to be susceptible to scientific quantifications and predictions. Who tries to count, compare and classify subjectivities? In their own way, perhaps, poets do so. Scientists do their best to avoid them.

Cancer has been associated with psychological states and personality types since the earliest times. The theory of humours laid out a number of detailed tie-lines between illness and psychological traits, linking cancer with an excess of the melancholy humour. This view was still maintained in the nineteenth century, though in a slightly refined form. Before 1900, as Lawrence LeShan pointed out in his speech at the Bristol Cancer Help Centre in November 1985, twenty-nine out of thirty medical textbooks associated the disease with suppressed emotion. This view was based on the accumulated observation of doctors over the centuries, but it fell victim to the twentieth century's enthusiasm for single causes in disease. By the 1920s, the connection between cancer and personality had all but dropped from the sight of the medical educators, though it continued as a prominent part of medical folklore. W. H. Auden expressed it in his popular ballad from the 1930s, 'Miss Gee', about the perils of sexual repression.

Doctor Thomas sat over his dinner
　　Though his wife was waiting to ring;
Rolling his bread into pellets,
　　Said: 'Cancer's a funny thing.

'Nobody knows what the cause is,
　　Though some pretend they do;
It's like some hidden assassin
　　Waiting to strike at you.

'Childless women get it,
　　And men when they retire;
It's as if there had to be some outlet
　　For their foiled creative fire.'

Auden, the son of a leading general practitioner, retained a fascination with medicine all his life. He may here have been quoting directly from his father, whose views (if they were his) would have been perfectly consistent with a doctor trained in the nineteenth century.

Yet to today's medicine, grounded in advanced technology, such imprecision – that 'nobody knows', 'it's as if' and 'cancer's a *funny* thing' – appears lame. The medical student is encouraged to find in the mechanical model of disease a more exciting career, with more confident explanations and more powerful procedures than those of Auden's tentative Dr Thomas. Such a doctor becomes a figure of fun, a Straw Man by comparison with the incisive Tin Men of medical technocracy, who now control the health services of all advanced nations, and increasingly of developing ones too. What this technocracy believes about cancer – one of its gravest problems – is, crudely, that self-as-mind *cannot* turn against self-as-body and generate the disease because (in Gilbert Ryle's terms) this is a logical absurdity, flying in the face of good scientific principles. This is today's orthodoxy. However, it is now beginning to be undermined from within the citadel of medicine itself. For a wind of change is emerging from the medical research laboratories, and it is blowing us nearer to the notion that personality, imagination, emotion and other subjective factors are, indeed, causal influences on the disease of cancer.

Cancer research and the personality

A first clue is that cancer is pre-eminently a human disease. It does exist among animals, but in the wild it is extremely rare. Indeed, the simpler the organism, the rarer tumours are. Is this a clue telling us that cancer has something to do with complexity, and in particular with sophisticated hormone, immune and nervous systems? Further clues come from seeing what happens when you try to induce cancer in animals: not a particularly pleasant field of research, but one from which a good deal has been learned. Typical of this research is that of Vernon Riley in Seattle. Working with cancer-prone strains in 1976, his team found that 60 per cent of heavily stressed rats got cancer, while only 7 per cent of unstressed ones did. The same team proved that isolated mice get cancer more quickly than those in 'normal-sized' social groups. Adult rats subjected to handling-stress also easily get cancer, but those which have been handled from a very young age are much more protected. Not only does cancer *start* more easily under stress, but tumours implanted into laboratory animals grow much more quickly, probably because of stress-lowered immunity – an effect I have already described.[4]

So animal studies do tend to support the stress link, but they have many drawbacks. Laboratory conditions in a rat's cage are not exactly most people's idea of a simulated human environment. Moreover, to surmount the difficulty of animal resistance to cancer, scientists must use special strains whose cancer resistance has been bred out of them. This is thus an artificial world whose association with the real one is speculative, therefore such research cannot shed much light on whether there is a particular type of human personality prone to cancer. In general, it seems to be as hard to induce cancer in people as in animals. In America – incredibly, one might think – long-term prisoners volunteered for a programme of research which involved their being injected with virulent cancer cells. This was found to cause local irritation only. The prisoners' defensive systems easily brushed the intrusive cells aside, although these were people in whom you would expect to find much stress.

So what makes cancer such a relatively common disease in humans? Perhaps there are certain kinds of human stress which make it more likely; or a particular type of personality which is more susceptible. The intuitive belief of most nineteenth-century doctors was that cancer comes out of a combination of the two. The disappearance of this consensus at the end of the Victorian age was followed by a new consensus centred around surgery. Following the invention and improvement of chemical anaesthesia, the surgeon now basked in all the glory due to glamourous 'action men' in the battle against disease. But the new prestige of surgical treatment fuzzed the issue, and the question 'How is the disease caused?' became obscured by the answer to another question: 'How shall we treat it?' And the answer of course was 'by surgery', followed by 'with radio-therapy' and today by 'with combined radio- and chemo-therapy'. Even forty years ago few significant medical authorities were prepared to maintain what looked like an obsolete non-mechanistic doctrine of causation in the face of such triumphantly established (though hardly triumphantly successful) modes of mechanical treatment.

This began to change in the early 1950s. Working in Glasgow with miners who had developed diseases of the lung, David Kissen gave these patients psychological tests before moving to a physical diagnosis. By looking for certain psychological characteristics, he found that he could predict which of the men would turn out to have cancer – rather than, say, pneumon-coniosis – in 70 or 80 per cent of cases. Arthur Schmale at the University of Rochester, N.Y., carried out similar tests on women who had entered hospital for cervical cancer biopsy. On the basis of his psychiatric examination alone, Schmale made a prediction as to whether these women had cancer. He then asked his medical team to conduct a general physical examin-ation (short of biopsy) and make their predictions. When the biosy was carried out, Schmale was right in 72.5 per cent of cases, while the medical team's average was no better than if they had tossed a coin.

So on what psychological characteristics were these predic-tions based? Kissen said he was looking for signs in the patient of *inadequate emotional outlet*, a criterion very similar to the one so frequently accepted a hundred years earlier. Schmale was also looking, in particular, for emotional withdrawal, self-containment and reserve.

LeShan, meanwhile, had picked up large-scale epidemiological hints connecting cancer with *loss*. From his own clinical experience – he is a psychotherapist – he was sure that emotional block or 'bottling up' was a significant risk factor for cancer. He further believed that such individuals would be particularly in danger of cancer if they lost a significant emotional relationship and could not replace it with an adequate substitute. If you divided people up by marital status, he reasoned, the ascending order of risk would be from the single, up through the married and the divorced and then to the highest risk group, the widowed. However, because of the many variables involved this effect would only be likely to be picked up by very large-scale, whole-population statistics. He reprints the following table in his book *You Can Fight For Your Life*:

Cancer mortality rates per 100,000 living population of the United States 1929–31, females only

	Breast	Uterus	Ovary, Fallopian tubes	Vulva and vagina	Other	Total
Single	15.0	9.0	3.3	0.5	33.4	61.2
Married	24.5	35.0	4.7	0.8	11.8	137.7
Divorced	29.3	57.2	6.0	1.5	81.8	175.8
Widowed	74.4	94.4	9.6	4.3	344.4	527.1

The obvious objection is that any disease whose incidence is higher in older people is more likely to happen to the widowed. But an English researcher quoted by LeShan looked at British government statistics for 1932 and found that widows *in all age groups* had a higher cancer mortality than the single or the married, and that 'the less satisfactory the marital status, the earlier the patient manifests cancer and dies from it.' LeShan also points out that another disease with a similar age-related mortality profile to that of cancer is diabetes, although the incidence of this is *not* greater in the widowed than in other women.

Evidence on the psychological profile of actual or potential cancer patients has emerged from John Hopkins Hospital in the United States. There, forty years ago, Caroline Thomas began a long-term study of a whole generation of medical students, first testing them psychologically and then following their health as it developed. When she looked back at the tests of those who later got cancer, she found there were definite common factors: a low-key non-aggressive personality, with repressed emotions and pronounced loneliness. These individuals were typically either not close to their parents, or had at some important point lost a parent to whom they were close – either through death or divorce.[6] Again, the theme of loss appears.

A comprehensive survey of all recent research in this area by two psychologists at the University of California[7] quotes study after study to confirm and elaborate LeShan's and Thomas's general themes. According to this summation of the three decades of research, the cancer personality seems to be centred round the same inability or unwillingness to express emotions, and to include the tendency to be passive in relationships and to defer to a partner. Other factors were sociability and 'niceness', industriousness, perfectionism, conventionality and defensiveness. The person who gets cancer is more likely to become resigned to adversity, and might thus be likely to have more invested in a stable (though perhaps unsatisfactory) marriage or relationship. He or she is also slightly less likely to suffer from depression. Cancer patients are classically *copers*. It is not a disease of people who go to pieces in face of stress, but rather of those who *hold themselves together too well*.

These are the outlines of the 'cancer personality' as it has been emerging from psychological research. But there is one further important finding, essentially a character trait and of crucial significance for the outlook for people with cancer. The less fatalistic and the more aggressive they are, the better their chance of recovering. LeShan sees a spiritual as well as a psychological similarity between people who get cancer. They have, he thinks, a Cartesian, mechanistic view of the world which leaves them badly equipped to fight this fight. 'Perceiving the cosmos as uncaring and unconcerned,' he says, 'the typical cancer patient does not conceive of any meaning beyond the human being and his particular relationship. Yet, at the same time, the individual has the feeling that he has been singled out by fate. No matter what he does, how hard he tries, the course of his life is seen as predetermined, joyless and doomed.' When this Cartesian pessimist meets the mechanisms of modern medicine, he sees a reflection of his own insignificance and is at an even greater disadvantage. Such is the spiritual outlook LeShan so often encounters, one of 'helplessness and hopelessness'.

These cancer patients described by LeShan were most often 'perfect' patients: compliant, passive, sweet-natured. Rarely did he find them truculent, angry and independent of mind, though those who were difficult usually did best. So the 'best' cancer patients are actually the worst ones, showing a fighting spirit and (perhaps) a contemptuous disregard for the gloomy forecasts of their doctors and relations. This opinion has been confirmed by work done in London by S. Greer at King's College Hospital in the 1970s. Greer's team found incontrovertible evidence that women with breast cancer who denied or fought their cancers had a much greater chance of recovery.[8] The significance of this last personality trait was brought home to me when I met Katarina Collins.

THE CASE OF KATARINA

I met Katarina during a visit to the Bristol Cancer Help Centre, where she is a voluntary unpaid counsellor. The help she gives there to hundreds of day-visiting cancer sufferers is doubly valuable because it is based on sound holistic principles and is derived almost entirely from her own experience. Several years ago, Katarina was diagnosed with breast cancer. She knew the facts of this disease and at first she went into a flat spin of panic. Now, looking back, she can see that her illness followed a classic pattern.

'I was a coper,' she said. 'I was very good at giving love, very good at cuddling. But I didn't know how to *ask* for love.' Katarina regarded herself as very happily married when suddenly she found her children growing up and her husband desperately ill with a long-drawn-out progressive illness. She nursed him for six years until he died. As I talked to her, one of the central ideas of this book came into perspective for me: illnesses which speak play variations on a single theme – they speak of loss, deprivation, incompleteness.

The amputee is tormented by phantom pains as his body protests against its lack. So, now, Katarina was a victim of a sudden and catastrophic emotional amputation. She had completely built herself around her family and its care, but now she found half of her was just not there any more, summarily chopped off like a hand or a leg. Her body's appalled response, she believes, was cancer.

Katarina was slow to realize that she could recover from the disease. Before anything could heal, she knew it was essential to *choose* life. When she did choose, she lost her fear and could set about rebuilding herself and her life. This involved a fierce transformation of diet, relationships and attitudes. It involved becoming hard and selfish, although Katarina was merely redressing a balance which had been skewed to one side for years. She needed to tap raw energy, to strip herself back to a raw state of being, so she ate raw food. She needed to rethink her life, so she gave herself time alone. She found it in herself to become demanding of love and emotion. Gradually her tumour, though it fought back, was put down and now she feels it is under control. Katarina does not feel 'cured', but she is now confident of being in control.

By the lights of any purely mechanistic biology, such effects do not occur. Katarina is simply 'lucky' – she just happens to be one of the roughly 50 per cent of breast cancer patients who do well, and she could probably have done well whatever her mental attitude. But Katarina simply *knows* this is untrue; she believes that by her own efforts she has slain a dragon, defeated rebellion and emerged in charge of her body and her life. The pathways and processes she used can so far only be guessed at, though they must involve the activation of the immune-system through the emotion-processing parts of the brain, including certainly the hypothalamus.

Katarina's path back to health is not everybody's. To seek *conventional* treatment is just as likely to express a determination to become well, and such determination undoubtedly will assist the effectiveness of that treatment. I highlight this case because it is a dramatic example of the influence of the patient's attitude: the effect already noticed by Greer and colleagues at King's. Human motivation is not a simple matter and it is not altogether surprising that doctors who specialize in cancer have so far fought shy of psychological factors, concentrating their efforts on surgical, radiological and chemical therapy. Yet we may have now reached a stage when these techniques are becoming self-limiting. The time is approaching when the role of the mind in cancer must be taken seriously.

In Susan Sontag's critique of the imagery surrounding cancer, she reserves much scorn for those who dramatize the 'war' against the disease with martial metaphors – 'bombardments' with X-rays, 'heroic' surgery, 'magic bullets' and the like. But such language is natural and I have used the image of a civil war for the same reason. Cancer *is* violence, a violence of the self against the self. Its association with frustration and unsatisfied desire and its spread with the increase of materialism does not look like an accident.

Lawrence LeShan[9] states that cancer patients 'always' have emotional elements missing from their lives. That, perhaps, is true of everyone. However LeShan looks in particular for the loss of *significant relationships for which no substitute has been found*. But, he says, the lack may go deeper than this; there may be a denial of the self, so that the lost significant relationship *may be with the self* – perhaps because of an 'excessive concern for the opinion of others'. This hostility towards the self is often, he says, expressed as the denial of some special talent or talisman which is felt to be of particular importance. To return to a relationship with oneself, it is necessary to 'sing your own song in your own way'. If LeShan is right, then cancer emerges as a personality disorder whose damaging effects are directed at the body. It then follows that though we may start with surgery, radiation, chemotherapy and the prevention of environmental hazards, the answer to cancer lies deeper. There is a proverb attributed to Jesus in the gnostic *Gospel of Thomas* which might have been written about cancer: 'If you bring forth what is within you, what you bring forth will save you. If you do not bring forth what is within you, what you do not bring forth will destroy you'.[10]

I conclude this chapter with a glance at a disparate group of non-cancerous diseases. These are not even remotely like cancer, except in so far as they are 'self against self' diseases and may have a rather similar emotional origin.

Auto-immunity

Auto-immune disease has been alternatively called 'auto-allergy' a name which, though a more descriptive term, has never quite caught on. Its mechanism is still a complete mystery, but to describe some of the best guesses let us return to antibodies and antigens. Every cell sports an antigen on its surface which, like a military cap-badge, identifies the unit to which the cell belongs. Thus my cells carry my personal antigen and yours display one peculiar to you. Identical twins having identical antigens have interchangeable cells, which means that tissue transplants between the two meet no rejection problems. Most transplant surgery, however, is utterly dependent on the doctor's ability to understand and suppress immune action against alien cells, using drugs like Azathioprine and Cyclosporin A. Any antigen in the body detected as alien by the individual's immune system automatically evokes antibodies which attack and deal with it in ways detailed in Chapter 5.

Auto-allergy is when antibodies are produced against one's own antigens, against the cells of Self. Usually it is confined to one organ or one type of tissue, as if the immunity police were possessed by some irrational prejudice against the cells of this or that system. Such treachery can only be explained in one of two ways: either there is a fault in the immune system itself – the production of rogue antibodies which see their job as roughing up law-abiding members of their own cell-society – or else some change has occurred in the antigens of these otherwise normal cells. Perhaps the cap-badges have been damaged, masked or somehow swapped with those of a genuine outsider.

It would be extremely helpful if the antigens themselves could be examined for clues as to which of these possibilities is correct. Unfortunately, no antigen has ever been seen; the word represents a hypothetical entity, or maybe just a molecular *shape*, whose differences are too small for even the finest electron microscope and whose characteristics may be as ineffable as the lineaments of a human face. So the existence of this show of individuality on the surface of cells has to be deduced from the fact that antibodies – which we *can* detect – do appear to recognize them. In the light of this difficulty, it is not altogether surprising that research into auto-immunity has made relatively little progress since the concepts underlying it were first outlined by the Australian Macfarlane Burnet and the Englishman Peter Medawar in the 1950s.

Yet there is plenty to discover here. One unpleasant disease in which auto-antibodies have been found – showing that auto-allergic changes have taken place – is ulcerative colitis. This is a severe chronic inflammation of the colon where the tender mucous membranes are apparently attacked and damaged by the immune system, leading to severe inflammation, secondary bacterial damage, chronic diarrhoea, bleeding and other complications. In the worst cases treatment is drastic, involving the surgical removal of the whole of the infected part (usually including the rectum) and the need to evacuate the gut via an ileostomy.

Some forms of anaemia are certainly auto-allergic – with the target 'auto-antigen' being the red blood cells. Another common disease in which auto-immunity is implicated is rheumatoid arthritis – a chronic inflammation in the body's connective tissue, especially the limb joints. It hits one person in twenty – but women are three times more prone – is extremely painful and disabling and there is no cure.

Diabetes too, especially when it appears in younger people, is increasingly seen as the possible result of auto-allergic damage in the pancreas, the insulin-producing gland. Another possible candidate is Addison's disease, a breakdown of the adrenal glands for which the cause is unknown in three out of four cases. So also is multiple sclerosis – another 'mystery disease' where under certain circumstances (perhaps following the presence of an unknown virus), antigens in the myelin sheaths covering the axons of nerve cells – like victims of mistaken identity – might perhaps be attacked as alien and permanently damaged. Other illnesses where auto-antibodies have been observed include thyroid, liver, skin and kidney diseases: conditions which forty years ago would never have been seen keeping the same company. Yet the concept of auto-immunity has completely changed the way in which these maladies are classified.

Many of them already have one other important factor in common: the mind. Every medical student knows that the emotions are associated with bowel disorders, but it is less widely appreciated that diabetes may be something to do with emotional and stressful states, as may arthritis, multiple sclerosis and Addison's disease. However, while the mechanism of auto-immunity remains so poorly understood, it is difficult to judge the plausibility of theories implicating the mind and emotions.

One of the difficulties is to tell whether the auto-antibody cells found in these conditions are a *cause* or a *result* of the disease process. Major errors can turn on mistaking a cause for an effect. For hundreds or even thousands of years, the belief that putrefying meat brought about the spontaneous generation of maggots was used to support the theory that lower life-forms arise of themselves out of non-living matter. It was not until 1668, when Francesco Redi excluded flies from rotten meat and observed no maggots, that putrefaction was seen as accidental to the process: a *cas*ual rather than a *caus*al link. If the presence of these auto-antibodies is merely a side-effect – even if an important one – of some viral infection, then links with the mind and the personality become somewhat weaker. If on the other hand, under the control of the hypothalamus the immune system is shown to be wantonly, destructively and spontaneously turning against the body's own cells, then we can begin to class these illnesses as psychosomatic. The research is still going on, particularly as a spin-off from the drive to control graft-rejection following transplants. However, the upshot may be to carry us far beyond the mechanistic world of spare-part surgery.

There is even some evidence of an 'auto-allergic' personality. G. F. Solomon looked at female arthritics and their healthy sisters to see if they differed psychologically from each other.[11] The common factor seemed to be the *renunciation or loss of independence*. These women were more liable to be compliant, masochistic, subservient, restless, depressed and repressed. They were also more likely to express extreme views on their husbands – either fulsomely to praise his consideration, or to portray him as a beast. Solomon believes these are the characteristics of an auto-immune personality, and gives the following illustrative case history.

THE CASE OF THE WOMAN RACING DRIVER

She was an army officer in her mid-thirties suffering from depression. Her life was tremendously active and independent; she was an avid sky-diver and one of the few women in international sports-car racing. In sport, her life thus depended on an unusual degree of perfectionism. However, when she wrecked her Maserati car she found the substitute inadequate; in Solomon's view, the loss of her beloved car combined with the frustrated search for perfection put her at risk. 'I felt that if anyone was likely to develop auto-immune disease it was she.' Looking at her medical history he found she had suffered from *purpura*, a blood-platelet disorder whose main symptom is a purple rash on the skin which was found to be of auto-immune origin. Three months later she came down with systemic *lupus erythematosus*, a chronic auto-immune disease of the connective tissue in which the skin erupts, the joints become painful and the kidneys, lungs and spleen are also affected. But this woman had clearly developed a 'disease which speaks', one that is also a disease of internal subversion, of self against self. Her case provides a very clear demonstration of the links between the immune system and psychological upset, at least in Solomon's view, although his description of the auto-immune personality must remain speculative.

Different though they are, cancer and auto-immune disease both present aspects of action by the self against the self. In both of them, too, we have encountered again the leitmotif of *loss* which seems to haunt so many psychosomatic illnesses.

As for the idea of personality types associated with cancer and auto-immune disease, these seem more in the way of sketches than detailed specifications. In spite of LeShan's extremely interesting work, it is obvious that human personality is naturally too various and quirk-ridden to be a fail-safe index of behaviour. I am sure he would agree with this. After all, the idea of putting people into categories so that you can then predict their behaviour is a totalitarian dream. Nevertheless, the indications and signposts towards people who may be cancer-prone – which is not the same thing as the disease being pre-ordained – are highly suggestive of a disease that is more than an unfortunate accident.

Chapter 7

The unconscious

'Freud took it upon himself to show us that
there are illnesses which speak – unlike
Hesiod, for whom the illnesses sent by Zeus
descended on mankind in silence.'
Jacques Lacan[1]

The notion of the unconscious ought to be indispensable to all
medicine, yet doctors concerned with organic disease almost
invariably behave as if it does not exist – or, at best, as if it does
not concern them. We have seen how the objective scientist
inevitably jibs at anything subjective. But perhaps another
reason for this lack of regard for the unconscious is its slightly
musty, museum-like connotations.

One of the drawbacks of the progressive view of science is a
dangerous susceptibility to crazes and fashions. This is not quite
like the to-and-fro movements of fashion in, for instance, the
style of clothes. Scientific fashions rarely look backwards, and
most medical crazes of the last two hundred years have long
since lapsed into the character of faintly ludicrous quaintness:
either ludicrously *obvious* ('the germ theory'), or ludicrously
passé (monkey-gland injections). Everything coming under the
spell of progressive fashion is thus destined to be refuted and
superseded, for nothing seems so unappealing in science as the
day-before-yesterday's fashion.

Following the inter-war period when it was extremely
fashionable, the unconscious was dismissed as a scientific curiosity, like one of those china busts for demonstrating phren-
ology. Yet, unlike phrenological bumps, the appeal of Freud's
theory of the unconscious mind never had anything to do with
its novelty. Freud knew that the unconscious has in some way
or another been recognized since antiquity. He constantly

emphasized that it is present in the pre-scientific explanations of myth, magic and religion, which his renegade disciple Jung took even more seriously. But despite Freud's own claim to scientific validity, such ideas do not attract doctors in a world of ever-updated clinical modernity.

Psychoanalysis has nothing to do with pushing the snowball of knowledge ever onwards. It is concerned with the inner and the hidden. The Egyptians and the Babylonians suspected that there are forces within us which work against our own superficial wishes and interests. They regarded different organs of the body, for example, as having powers which the person as a whole had great difficulty in bringing under conscious control. Plato's account of the reproductive parts gave them particularly mischievous powers, indeed an autonomy which amounts to having a mind of their own:

A man's genitals are naturally disobedient and self-willed, like a creature that will not listen to reason, and will do anything in their mad lust for possession. Much the same is true of the matrix or womb in women, which is a living creature within them which longs to bear children. And if it is left unfertilised long beyond the normal time, it causes extreme unrest, strays about the body, blocks the channels of the breath and causes in consequence acute distress and disorders of all kinds. This goes on until the woman's longing and the man's desire meet and pick the fruit from the tree, as it were, sowing the ploughland of the womb with seeds as yet unformed and too small to be seen, which take shape and grow within until they are born into the light of day as a complete living creature.[2]

Rubbing the dust off this, it comes up rather fresh. Despite being utterly, even disastrously wrong in factual detail, it has a certain truth in suggesting this second order of mind at work in me, independent of the Mind which I am used to thinking of as 'Me'. However, this conscious Mind is the public 'Me' only. It co-exists with a private 'Me' whose effect is often to cut across my public performance and produce performances of its own. These performances may be not merely exploitations of physical states, such as the kind of psychological control of hormones discussed in the last chapter; they may go further into the *creation of* disease states themselves.

In this chapter I shall examine disease as performance in its most well-known form, hysteria – the ability of the mind to create organic symptoms which are indistinguishable from those caused by the 'genuine' disease. As we shall see, hysteria is less often recognized today; doctors, like patients, are not inclined to see it as 'real', so it has become like a ghost which in our fear we hope not to see at all. But hysteria *is* real and ever with us. Today it wears a variety of constantly changing disguises.

It is hardly surprising that the ancients located the origin of this condition – regarded as a wholly female complaint – in the reproductive organs. The last chapter made it clear how the complex of desires and fears surrounding reproduction can have a material effect on the body of an individual. Hysteria was once thought to be an entirely internal matter, the consequence of the same 'wandering womb' to which Plato refers. In fact, though it may today be classified as a psychological illness, it cannot be regarded as private or personal at all. Hysteria is above all an acknowledgement that we are social beings; it is a social disease, a public event.

But to understand this we need to look again at sex, this time from the viewpoint of the social and psychological climate in which people live and grow.

The myth of female wickedness

The story of the womb teaches us more than the scientific history of any other organ (including the brain) about the power of superstition in society, and in the medicine which society sanctions and practices. For thousands of years the womb has enclosed and embodied the male's paranoia about the female, which is probably the most significant collective male neurosis. 'Women have very little idea how much men hate them', says Germaine Greer.[3] But before they hate, people generally fear; before they fear, they generally desire; and before they can desire, there must be a separated *object* to be desired. In so far, then, as she is seen as 'other' by the male, the female is – in one way or another – the object of his desire and thus of his fear: a source of simultaneous fascination and repulsion.

On the primeval fantasy of female wickedness has been hung the whole apparatus of patriarchal control in public and family life. Historically, the woman's reproductive processes, the autonomic and cyclical actions of her womb, were matters of great psychological, social and economic consequence to the man, since without them how could he reproduce himself? But as reproduction was a matter which he did not understand and could not control, the biology of women became a bogey, an imaginary plexus of pollutions and fearful mysteries whose fearfulness increased exactly in proportion to their importance. In Chapter 3 I mentioned the deeply ingrained link between *fear* and *impurity*. An enormous body of lore and custom arose from this image of women's insides, which regarded menstruating women and new mothers as unclean. The exclusion of the new mother from Christian Sunday services until she is 'churched' (or purified) survived into this century, and is still practised by fundamentalist groups.

D. H. Lawrence is a modern writer who, for feminists, has come to epitomize the snarling Dobermann beneath the courteous skin of patriarchy. His attitude to the gynaecological mystery is anything but modern, as can be gleaned from one of his most peculiar poems called 'Figs'.

> There was a flower that flowered inward, womb-ward;
> Now there is a fruit like a ripe womb.
> It was always a secret.
> That's how it should be, the female should always
>   be secret . . .
> Fig, fruit of the female mystery, covert and inward,
> Mediterranean fruit, with your covert nakedness
> Where everything happens invisible, flowering and
>   fertilising, and fruiting
> In the inwardness of your you, that eye will never see
> Till it's finished, and you're over-ripe, and you burst
>   to give up your ghost . . .

This may be more than a little ridiculous, but it hardly conceals its sexual excitement, a combination of wonder, fear and disgust. In *Lady Chatterley's Lover*, Lawrence's attitude to the male genitals – or at least, to those of the gamekeeper Mellors – is strikingly similar to that of Plato. 'John Thomas' is regarded as a character, a person in its own right, very wilful and impulsive. It is distinct from the attitude of the man to whom it is attached, for the man – if we take Mellors as a stand-in, or stunt-man for Lawrence – lacks the sexual straightforwardness of his own penis. As the critic Kate Millett pointed out, Lawrence's ecstatic full-frontal celebrations of the male member are nowhere matched in his presentation of the woman's body. 'Although the male is displayed and admired so often,' says Millett, 'there is, apart from the word cunt, no reference to or description of the female genitals; they are hidden, shameful and subject'.[4] Lawrence's negative feelings about the female sexual anatomy are certainly on display in 'Figs', in particular at the poem's questioning, nervous conclusion:

> Ripe figs won't keep, won't keep in any clime.
> What then, when women the world over have all bursten
>   into self-assertion?
> And bursten figs won't keep?

It was from this type of neurosis, primitive yet remarkably and disturbingly persistent into our own times, that flowed all the taboos about menstruation, all the myths about witchcraft, even the complex of ingrained beliefs surrounding macho man and the *femme fatale* which have been used over the millennia to build a barrier between the sexes.

In the past the outward signs of hostility were more pronounced. Women were sometimes treated little better than lepers – segregated, excluded, regarded as diseased and impure in their very natures. They had to be employed, yes, but wherever possible a distance was maintained publicly between them and their menfolk. They ate apart, prayed apart, worked separately. This happen in parts of our world today. We are familiar with the ritual segregation of women in mosques and synagogues, but among Armenian Christians in Turkey – a wealthy and educated community – men and women still worship in different parts of the church. And in case anyone should imagine such practices are safely in the historical or geographical far distance, I have met in Ireland an old couple who, in the privacy of their simple life together, illustrated the syndrome starkly. In that cottage he ate his meals always alone, at the table, while she took her food apart on a low stool beside the fire. Perhaps they could not have said why they did this, beyond the fact that they always had.

Meanwhile, countless working men's clubs all over Britain

systematically exclude or separate women. At the other end of the social scale, the headquarters of the Royal Yacht Squadron at Cowes in the Isle of Wight has a separate staircase used by women. Peasants, urban proletariat and elite – all are inheritors of the same neurosis.

The legacy of centuries leaves its mark on women's attitudes to their bodies, so the medical assumption – which is historically conventional – that women are more prone than men to psychosomatic illnesses is not surprising. Plato thought that 'the men of the first generation who lived cowardly or immoral lives were, it is reasonable to suppose, reborn in the second generation as women'.[5] Just to be a woman was a punishment, and it has already been noted with reference to pain that a sense of guilt can prompt the mind to create disease. The most baffling of all such disease syndromes is hysteria – a condition considered through the centuries to be exclusively female and so named after the womb, which in Greek is *hystera*.

The wilful womb

In common parlance, hysteria is a particular type of inappropriate behaviour, such as uncontrollable outbursts of laughter at a funeral, or convulsions and fainting after some frightening experience. It is still usually regarded as something done by women, not men. 'Hysterical pregnancy' is also widely known about and is obviously a female complaint, though men do feel 'sympathetic labour pains', presumably by similar mechanisms to those discussed in Chapter 3. The reality of this fascinating clutch of symptoms and somatic events is rather more complicated than common parlance would suggest.

The first known clinical descriptions of hysteria were by Egyptian doctors almost 4,000 years ago. The oldest medical writings we have from ancient Egypt detail bizarre female behaviour and symptoms, which were put down to the migration of the womb within the body's cavity. Treatment was a carrot-and-stick affair: fumigation of the woman's sexual parts with fragrant smokes to lure the adventuring organ back to base, or else the use of disgusting potions down the throat in the hope of repelling it back.

This notion was taken over entirely by the Greeks and, via

the doctrines of Hippocrates and Galen, was transmitted into the medicine of the Christian West. Since then the history of hysteria has largely consisted in the narrowing down and refinement of the disease's definition and the search for a more plausible physical cause. So, does hysteria exist? Quite obviously the womb can no longer be regarded as some kind of bat which goes flapping around the peritoneum when disturbed. Nevertheless, the condition supposedly caused by these flights of panic has been repeatedly described and its basket of symptoms exhaustively itemized, notably by the great French neurologist Charcot in the 1880s. A fanatical observer of clinical data, it was he who finally shattered any remaining theoretical connections between hysteria and the uterus.

Charcot was following in the tradition of investigative physicians like the Englishmen Thomas Sydenham and Thomas Willis who both found hysteria fascinating, not least because it had varied physical symptoms, was especially common among younger people and had no known cause. Even when you strip away diseases which we now know to have a separate identity (such as Huntingdon's chorea and multiple sclerosis), there is still plenty of evidence that the illness these men were occupied with was a distinct disease, although of an infuriatingly elusive nature.

Sydenham's description of hysteria's clinical signs was particularly intelligent and stands up remarkably well today. He was a rationalist and a Cartesian mechanist and in tackling this subject, which he claimed accounted for no less than one-sixth of all diseases, he may have partly wanted to subvert surviving Medieval superstitions about witchcraft and demonic possession. So for him, hysteria was what today might be called a 'life-style' disease, coming not from some external 'possession' but as a result of profound internal disturbances connected with the patient's mode of life. He stated that it was nothing whatever to do with the womb and in fact was not even confined to women, since in his view hypochondria in men was an identical syndrome.

As to its symptoms, these were bewildering. Sydenham distinguished two forms of the disease, one of which comes close to the popular notion of hysterical behaviour where the patient twitches uncontrollably, has head pains and throat constrictions (*globus hystericus*) and may vomit, faint or laugh and cry uninhibitedly. However, he also described another form of hysteria – which was perhaps the same form but unrecognized until then – whose repertoire of symptoms had a virtually unlimited range from false pregnancy to actual death. If 'classical' hysteria can be said broadly to imitate the signs of epileptic and apoplectic fits, this wider definition allows the simulation of any symptom. As Sydenham says: 'Of all the affections that poor mortals suffer, there is not one that cannot be imitated by hysteria'.[6] This is an observation which he made not from the academic text of his time – Galen – but from his patients themselves, and it goes right to the heart of the disease. The ability to *mimic* is the hallmark of hysterical phenomena, the puzzle which would always bring it to the attention of great neurological thinkers such as Charcot and Freud. It is also the reason why hysteria is central to this book: above all conditions acknowledged by medical science, this proclaims the ability of Mind to make things happen to Body, exactly as if they had been done by *another* Body – a falling solid object, a microbe (unknown of course in Sydenham's day) or another human being's violent action.

Sydenham guessed that there were two sides to the physical life of humanity, an *exterior* and an *interior*, of which the former was the visible anatomy while the latter contained a grid of powerful but invisible forces. This 'inner man' is not the psyche – Sydenham was too much the follower of Descartes for that – but it stands proxy for the psychic principles which Freud would later deploy to such effect. It amounts to a kind of interior force-field which, Sydenham tells us, is:

composed of the necessary concatenation of the spirits, arranged in some sort of structure, and observable only in the light of reason. Intimately connected with the life of the body, and joined, as it were, to it, the 'inner man' is more or less easily unsettled depending on the lesser or greater natural firmness of our constituent principles.[7]

These efforts to bring reason to bear on the question of the 'inner human being' – a challenge which was Freud's project, too – did little to counter the ignorance and fear which continued to dominate the subject of female ill-health, and ill-health generally, throughout the seventeenth, eighteenth and nineteenth centuries. The eighteenth century, the 'age of reason', was in particular and inevitably fascinated with and terrified of unreason. Some idea of the savagery of this climate can be formed from a reading of Michel Foucault's great study *Madness and Civilisation.* Foucault describes how the balance of medical opinion on hysteria gradually tilted towards purely mental explanations during the eighteenth century, and how these became increasingly moral and punitive.

Such changes in intellectual fashion meant that eventually organic and mental illness would go their separate ways. Then came the psychiatric specialist such as Philippe Pinel, working in France in the early nineteenth century. Pinel believed he could demonstrate that the physical symptoms (the 'mimicry') of hysteria could not be accounted for by any physical changes in either brain or nervous system. Pinel's model of hysteria in women was strikingly similar to the concept of 'learned pain behaviour' which was examined in Chapter 2 and whose treatment was 'eliminating the rewards resulting from pain behaviour and substituting more active and constructive behaviours'. Pinel adopted a similar approach to mental patients; since he saw them as having somehow become removed from the magic circle of morally acceptable behaviour, he aimed to return them to normal functioning primarily through sermons, marriage and purposeful work. So, while on the face of it Pinel's asylum in Paris was a model of enlightened humanity, behind its kindly façade was a prototype 'total institution', where patients were assessed on their record of co-operation. It is easy to see why in this century he has been hailed as the first true psychiatrist.

Vapours

Such moralistic views were congenial to the men of the nineteenth century, especially as they were then witnessing an upsurge in female hysterical illness unprecedented since the witchcraft scares of two centuries earlier. In general, the Victorian age was inauspicious for female mental health. Deeply repressed sexually and emotionally, and with social and material conditions changing rapidly as industrialization created more aggressive class divisions, bourgeois women in particular found themselves hedged around by new moral and social restrictions. These conditions demanded a 'modernized' role for the woman without changing her sexual inferiority, and in a psychological sense that must have been deeply stressful. Indeed, the surprising thing is not that a climate of repressed hostility between men and women was created, but that it remained repressed for so long – and in fact probably remains largely at that level to this day.

What appears to have happened in the Victorian age was a virtual epidemic of hysterical illnesses. It was as if a silent guerrilla movement, using pathology as a weapon, was sweeping through Europe with the all-male medical profession an obvious prime target. The doctors' response was occasionally harsh and the classical treatment would be that of Pinel: domesticity and subjection to the right type of husband, if available. But for intransigent cases, surgical operations might be prescribed: removal or cauterization of the ovaries or even, in cases of extreme punitive zeal, of the clitoris. The fact that these men – who called themselves scientists – directed their scalpels straight towards a woman's reproductive and sexual organs shows that their real inspiration came from superstitions that were older that the pharaohs.

On the surface, of course, most women in the last century accepted the verdicts of medicine, but this made them all the more likely to reproduce the essentially passive pattern of imitative hysterical illness – the type of weaknesses 'expected of them'. The most common hysterical symptom was quite different from the convulsive excesses of hysteria in the Middle Ages. Now it largely assumed the form of 'the vapours'. These were survivors of the belief in humoural fluids – harmful exhalations from the organs, originally the womb, but in popular and polite Victorian currency usually transferred to the stomach. It was a nebulous but – among the upper and middle classes – almost universally fashionable condition which involved flushes, fainting and depression, and seems obviously based on the very real physiological effects of menstruation, pregnancy and menopause.

Where the people could hardly afford doctors but relied instead on folk beliefs, a set of much older and more primitive and less sanitized medical ideas still held sway. Middle-class Europe may have rationalized the primeval misogyny into a

151

system of spurious scientific morality, but the peasants had hardly changed at all. Women in parts of Germany continued to believe that the uterus was a frog or some other animal, whose jumps and wanderings were the cause of their internal aches and pains.[8] But either way, the upshot was much the same: the diagnosis of hysteria meant that women could be denied the freedom of action which men took for granted. In some cases, if men preferred to have it both ways at once, women could be regarded as *willing* victims of their own moral and bodily weakness.

Charcot – Breuer – Freud

Charcot, a scientist so famous that he enjoyed all the prestige of an Einstein in his lifetime, hoped to demythify hysteria by demonstrating that it was a genuine neurosis and not a learned pattern of behaviour. However, his views on neurosis were strictly mechanical. He regarded hysterics as people – male or female – with a hereditary degeneration of the brain that is tripped into symptoms by some trauma. There was also a supposed link with hypnosis, which could be used to simulate hysterical symptoms such as paralysis, pains and anaesthesias.

When Sigmund Freud went to Paris during the winter of 1885–6 as an ambitious young neurologist, it was to sit at the feet of this great man whose ideas on hysteria he found particularly challenging. 'But he engrosses me', Freud wrote home excitedly. 'When I go away from him I have no more wish to work at my own simple things. My brain is sated as after an evening at the theatre. Whether the seed will ever bring forth fruit I do not know. But what I certainly know is that no other human being has ever affected me in this way'.[9] In fact, the seed fruited in due course into psychoanalysis, the most far-reaching psychological theory in history.

Freud's life's work – in Jacques Lacan's summary, that of illuminating the reality of 'maladies which speak' – did not begin until he worked on hysteria. Hysterical symptoms, Freud argued, were communications from an unconscious mind whose nature he could as yet only begin to glimpse. A disagreeable experience or an uncomfortable insight is suppressed from the memory, only to resurface insistently but in coded form as a physical symptom. Thus crude behaviourist methods of correction are useless; even if you can silence the symptom, another one will surely take its place. The only lasting treatment was somehow to retrieve the meaning of the symptoms by recalling, reprocessing and disposing of the initial experience or perception. But how could this be done?

Even before he met Charcot, Freud had become friendly with Josef Breuer, a Viennese doctor who had experimented with hypnotism for some time. Like Charcot, he had used trance states to study and treat hysterics, although he was ultimately to assist Freud in forming some quite opposite conclusions about the condition. The most puzzling of Breuer's cases was to provide a keynote case history to the two friends' epoch-making book *Studies in Hysteria*.

THE CASE OF FRAULEIN ANNA O.

Breuer was called in when Anna, an intelligent young woman of twenty-one, collapsed through exhaustion whilst nursing her fatally ill father to whom she was devoted. As soon as she was forced to leave her father's bedside, her exhausted state at once became exacerbated by a persistent cough. New symptoms then began to accumulate alarmingly: extreme tiredness, sleep-walking, a squint, visual disturbances, paralysis of the right arm and neck later spreading to the left side, so that eventually she could only turn her head by hunching her shoulders and rotating her whole trunk.

Next Breuer noted a curious speech disturbance. 'She was at a loss to find words. Later she lost her command of grammar and syntax,' he reports. Soon she was speaking in pigeon-German, until even this ability deserted her. When her paralysis slightly improved she suddenly regained the power of speech, but to her doctor's surprise 'she spoke only in English – apparently, however, without knowing she was doing so. She would have disputes with her nurse who was, of course, unable to understand her.' When her 'adored father' died, things became even worse. She had daytime hallucinations 'full of terrifying figures, death's heads and skeletons', which were followed in the evenings by trance-like states during which she would mumble disconnectedly to herself. Breuer found that if, during these auto-hypnotic episodes Anna could be persuaded to recount the contents of her day's hallucinations, she would then become much clearer and happier. It was what she referred to as her 'talking cure' – a phrase which was to resonate through the entire story of psychoanalysis.

A breakthrough came when Anna developed a sudden attack of screaming hydrophobia. For three days she was completely unable to drink water until, under hypnosis, she remembered her surge of disgust at seeing a dog lap from a glass of water intended for human consumption. As soon as this recollection appeared, the hydrophobia vanished. Breuer acted on the hints from Anna's own 'talking cure' and from the suppressed and salvaged memory of the lapping dog. He began a game of hide-and-seek with Anna's symptoms, tracing them patiently back to their origins first by taking notes of her auto-hypnotic ramblings, then by hypnotizing her himself. One by one Breuer extracted the symbolic meanings in each of Anna's symptoms and no sooner were they articulated than they disappeared.

For Breuer, the Anna O. incident had a highly unsatisfactory outcome. The patient developed a violent passion for her doctor – a phenomenon which Freud would later enshrine in psycho-analytical lore as 'transference' – and this scared the timorous Breuer almost out of his skin. No doubt smarting from his own guilty feelings in case he might have encouraged her, he abandoned the case.

When Freud heard all about this from a friend, it fascinated him. His subsequent study of hysteria – at first in collaboration with Breuer – was the starting point which turned him away from physiology and towards psychotherapy, away from a simple mechanistic view of mental function to a profoundly different one based on the notion of interplay between conscious and unconscious. That is a story which does not need to be repeated in detail here. However, the psychoanalytic model of mind was so revolutionary and became so influential that it is necessary to rehearse it briefly.

Freud believed that we are all neurotic in our natures. This is because the instincts of individual satisfaction clash with the requirements of collective survival. The 'ego instincts', which for Freud were largely crude sexual feelings, are therefore firmly repressed, but they return to us via the symbolic language of dream experience. If this is insufficient to discharge the repressed tension, they may then break into waking life as psychosomatic symptoms or disturbed behaviour, at which point they become pathological.

Freud was enough of a physiologist to realize that eventually many of the psychosomatic mechanisms would be discovered: in fact, he predicted rightly that these would be largely chemical. But his insistence that mind is like an ocean with some of its creatures flitting around near the surface, while the rest live hidden in the deeps, has created a first platform for dynamic opposition to the behaviourist-reductionist model of human nature. Yet behaviourists, with their easy answers to all the problems of education, economics and health, still effectively control our industrialized lives. To governments and other power-brokers, reductionism is so convenient; the implications of psychoanalytical thinking are so uncomfortable.

Hysteria now

It loomed so very large in the medical life of the nineteenth century, yet hysteria seems to have been almost struck from the list of 'Approved Diseases' today. Ilza Veith, the historian of the disease,[10] suggests that Freud himself, having laid bare the hysterical process, rendered it no longer possible for a patient to use hysteria as a ploy for obtaining psychological purchase on doctors and others. In the same way, a magician's most amazing illusions look transparent once you have seen how it was done with mirrors. But hysterical neurosis is much more than a trick, although it is often caricatured as such. No neurosis is so simple.

The reason for the apparent disappearance of this condition is partly avoidance of the word itself, if not of the idea. It carries so many pejorative connotations that its use has grown rare and reluctant. Writing in The Lancet, a professor of medicine has speculated about the effects of letting patients see their own medical notes, among which he thought they would come across 'apparently insulting or objectionable statements' – of which 'hysteria' was given as an example.[11] Both patients and doctors show extreme distaste for the diagnosis, preferring what they hope to be a more 'real' – by which they mean a more mechanical – illness.

There is, however, another reason for the 'disappearance':

the protean nature of the syndrome itself. The mythical Proteus, King of Pharos – an island off Egypt – shares so many features with the disease we have been discussing that it might well be renamed 'Proteus disease'. He was a sea-king, the 'first minister to Poseidon' who according to the *Odyssey*, 'knew the unplumbed ocean-pits'; hysteria, too, inhabits the unplumbed ocean depths of the unconscious mind. Proteus was an oracle, consulted for his insight and ability to articulate what is masked or garbled; hysteria, as I have already said, is one of the 'illnesses which speak'. But Proteus' most notable feature is his bewildering ability to change shape – originally, says Robert Graves in *The Greek Myths*, 'to mark the seasons through which the sacred king moved from birth to death'; hysteria has also constantly altered its 'shape' through the seasons of historical change.

In ancient times it was normally a malaise, characterized by depression and lethargy. When the witch-hunting craze was at its peak in the Middle Ages, hysteria took on the form of violent convulsions and screaming because these resembled demonic 'possession'. By the nineteenth century, such convulsive behaviour had given way to the more gentle, more ladylike but more chronic 'vapours'. As *the* fashionable female complaint of the Victorian era, the vapours chimed faithfully with the approved image of woman's delicate ethereal nature. So what of today? Today we have new words. The Department of Health and Social Security's *Social Security Statistics*[12] on absenteeism from work in Britain, for instance, record that in the course of the 1970s the instances of people excusing themselves from work on the grounds of 'symptoms and ill-defined conditions' increased by 23 per cent among men and no less than 50 per cent among women. Perhaps instead of 'possession', instead of the 'vapours', we should read 'symptoms and ill-defined conditions', although the usual medical term would be 'functional' illness.

There is, however, one condition which has very clearly come to the fore in the past fifteen years, and is obviously related to hysteria. Like the 'vapours' in the nineteenth century, this is a disorder which has accommodated itself to the public conception of a desirable woman in the second half of the twentieth century.

Anorexia has always been an element in hysteria (Anna O. suffered from it), though it was rarely heard of outside medical jargon until about twenty years ago. Now, of course, it is a household phrase. Anorexia is a classic conversion neurosis, taking its form from powerful social images – the fashion trends exemplified by jogging and by string-bean, asexual fashion models. Its mechanism is switched on somewhere in the hypothalamus, the centre of so many life-dependent processes: emotion, appetite control, sexuality. In anorexia all three are implicated and like three weird sisters, they make fair seem foul and foul seem fair, for sufferers can rarely accept that they are inflicting a grotesque emaciation on their bodies.

Anorexia is a very serious disease which in 10 per cent of cases results in death. Its 'trigger is often an extreme family situation, the death of a parent or an engagement to marry about which the patient is ambivalent'.[13] It is pre-eminently an 'illness which speaks', as the following thumbnail sketch of its course indicates.

It usually begins with dieting in adolescent girls, although at that time of hormonal change it is natural to carry 'puppy fat'. Dieting is such a 'normal' activity that over three stone can be shed without much family concern, by which time the syndrome has taken an unshakable grip. The hormones themselves are radically disturbed and appear to support the patient's denial of her sexual maturity; the male hormone testosterone increases, as does the female hormone oestriol; but the *main* hormones of the mature female – oestrone and oestradiol – become much harder to find in the blood. As this happens, the breasts disappear while the underarm and pubic hair falls out. Yet such is the disturbance to the patient's body-image that she continues to see in the mirror the fat woman she does not want to be.

She now begins to exhibit the painful brittleness of someone starving to death. If you force-feed her, she vomits. The sight and smell of food, especially fat and carbohydrate, seem especially nauseous. She feels driven to jog or otherwise to take massive doses of exercise. She suffers from insomnia, but strangely this is welcomed; unlike the depressive, she does not long for sleep. Aggressively she asserts throughout that she is feeling fine.

By the time her weight has sunk to that of a five-year-old, her immune system has collapsed and she begins to pick up opportunistic infections such as pneumonia and tuberculosis. When finally she dies, it is from such infection, if not from starvation.[14]

As this makes clear, anorexics can regress to a state before puberty – the weight 'of a five-year old', the abolition of sexual characteristics, the pathetic dependency merging with defiant assertions of independence. Sufferers will find recovery a hard road unless someone can help them to read the oracular message the disease is delivering.

I have dwelt at length on 'Proteus disease' because its history is also to a large extent that of clinical medicine. Wherever great advances have been made, hysteria seems to have featured in the literature: in the first clinical writings from Egyptian medicine; in Cos with the early Hippocratic scientists; in Plato and Galen; at the Renaissance, when all the great and famous doctors of medicine grappled with it; in the development of nineteenth-century psychiatry and neurology; and at the very inception of psychoanalysis. Only in our own time, when the unconscious is medically disregarded and 'illnesses which speak' go persistently unheard, has hysteria fallen from view.

Chapter 8

Instress

'In the final analysis human life is lived to
die, a pre-planned suicide, a chronic death
by voodoo'
Alfred Ziegler, Jungian psychologist[1]

A large proportion of medical resources is spent on death –
investigating it and looking for ways of reducing its occurrence.
In fact death itself is not a problem; of all natural processes, it
is the most perfectly comprehensible.

All organisms live permanently on a razor's edge of extinction. Their very existence is bought with a loan from nature,
the advance of the energy necessary to maintain the patterned
chemistry of life just long enough to reproduce. This has been
described as the dream of every cell: to become two cells.[2] But
sooner or later every organism, every cell must default on the
mortgage it has taken out. Then the minute net of molecules
which make that cell, and the intertwined society of cells which
makes that organism, begin to pull themselves apart string by
string. This process of *entropy* is the tendency of all physical
systems towards disorganization, decreed by the second Law
of Thermodynamics. Life exists in defiance of entropy, keeping
the tide at bay for a time like a sand-castle's wall. Reproduction,
the project of biology, is a principle of extension, prolonging
the system's existence beyond the life-span of the individual
unit. But in the end, the debt must still be paid: darkness and
chaos shall inevitably inherit the universe and there is nothing
any of us can do about it.

However, when the tide threatens to flood the banks of a
great river, the intellectual challenge is not in the nature of
water or of wetness, but in maintaining adequate tidebanks and
an effective barrier to keep it at bay. So, with mortality, the

question is not, 'What is death and why do we die?' but, 'What defines life and how do we stay alive?'

Life is not just energy, since energy exists without life. But life is energy in a particular container, energy restrained and channelled as if for a purpose. Life is that which knows what to do with energy, how to capture and direct it. The essence of the containment of energy is found in the word 'stress'.

Anyone who has ever erected a tent knows the principle. The tent collapses unless it is put under stress from guy-ropes – a stress which must be in balance, setting up a tied tug-of-war at the centre of which is perfect stability. We have already seen how self-regulating systems like pain-gates and hormone-controls maintain the balancing acts of the human biology. Life's ability to generate stress through energy is its foundation. The word which for me best captures this idea was coined by the Victorian poet Gerard Manley Hopkins 120 years ago: *instress*.

Instress referred to the quality which all objects (organic and inorganic) need in order to maintain their 'inscape', their distinctiveness. It also identified a mental or spiritual experience of that distinctiveness by the observer – in effect, a line of communication between mind and nature. Really there is no difference between the two aspects of instress, since what excited Hopkins about it was that it revealed nature (reality, creation) as fundamentally a web of interdependence and variegation: 'Glory be to God,' he wrote, 'for dappled things!'

'All things are upheld by instress and are meaningless without it,' he wrote elsewhere.[3] Tents attain and maintain their shape by virtue of the guy-ropes which are braced against the ground, but they cannot exist at all without inherent instress; the tent is nothing without the rigidity of the tent-poles, the tensile strength of the canvas and ropes. Now consider a free-floating soap bubble. Here the stress (surface tension) is utterly integral: practically, it *is* the bubble, so that when it is lost the bubble bursts and ceases to exist. Life is the maintenance of this kind of instress in cells. All things depend to some degree on outstress; but instress is a principle within living nature.

Another word for it which is fashionable at the moment is morphogenesis, the creation and maintenance of form in nature. Living organisms constitute the most highly patterned forms, physically so complex that they defy comprehension. Humanity adds a further dimension of complexity, that of thought and emotion, which are morphogenetically protean since they consist in much change and interchange of instress and outstress. Taken as a whole, the system of the human body is remarkably invariant and stable, trading between instress and outstress as efficiently as a well-run marketplace; yet, unless balanced, outstress can threaten the body's integrity and if this happens for long, instress – the positive principle of integrity – loses its purchase, slackens. If that occurs in a living structure, collapse and death sooner or later will follow.

Instress is a unitary and holistic concept. It is not only a physical attribute but a mental and spiritual quality too, although to put it like that seems to imply divisions between the physical, psychological and spiritual which do not in reality exist. Where instress exists in the body, it must be there also in the mind and the spirit. When instress is destroyed – whether in the mind, the body or the soul – it inevitably destroys the whole.

Consider death by suggestion. We have already considered in detail how physiological symptoms can be conjured by auto-suggestion in the hysteric. These are usually represented as superficial and not life-threatening, since the mind-body is supposedly employing a strategy for its advantage and not its destruction. However, it is part of the thesis of this book that self-destruction (as Freud knew) may easily become the object of the unconscious mind, and that psychosomatic self-injury is a common way of achieving this.

Another starting point might be the witch-doctor's ability to destroy instress, to commit psychic murder.

Witch-death

In the British Solomon Islands well into this century – and despite all the armies of straw-hatted Christian soldiers which moved in to combat him – the activities of the vellayman still struck dread into the hearts of the people. In a BBC radio programme in 1986, a missionary remembered:

The vellayman is someone who has this power, but nobody knows who he is, and he has everybody in awe of him. He would make

161

a noise in the bush, and we would hear this at night, and the boys would say (in a whisper) 'There's a vellayman out.'

He has a little bag of leaves and earth, and he would meet somebody in the bush, and hold this bag hanging from his finger, his arm stretched out, and they would know what it was and be terrified.

And he'd say to them you will go back to the village, and you'll not remember who I am, but you will know you are going to die in so-many days. So they would go back, and they wouldn't remember, and they *would* die.

One of the schoolboys said that he had once been attacked by a vellayman, and had lived to tell the tale. He said he was saved because he had vomited. And what I believe the vellayman does is make people eat whatever it is they have in the bag, and it is this that kills them.[4]

Deaths similarly caused by the remote exercise of human malice can be found in anthropological writings about primitive people the world over. But this particular witness has almost certainly heavily simplified the process, since the killing of a person by magic is never a casual act as it seems to be here. If it were, why not leap out from behind a tree and crush the victim's head with a stone instead? To be effective, a sorcerer must normally make many stylized and very complicated ritual preparations. The bag would be prepared in a specific way, especially for the purpose of attacking this particular victim.

The Kai, an inland people of the north-east part of New Guinea, practise a comparable witchcraft but incredibly elaborated. First, the victim's soul-stuff – some piece of his body, or anything touched by him – is placed as the nucleus of a packet made of leaves and bamboo, assembled over several days and kept apart in a hut of special design raised on ground known to be haunted. During this time, the sorcerer chants incantations to the giant lizards and the cockatoo, drawing down curses: 'Let X disappear in pains. May his limbs writhe in pains. May his whole body writhe in pains. May his entrails be contracted in pains. May his genitals be twisted in pains.' At the end of this long series of ceremonies, a number of other sorcerers are summoned to a feast in that same haunted place. These are then assigned parts and, in a remarkable piece of ritual theatre, the victim's demise is enacted in scenes so detailed as to include his relatives and friends arguing across the death-bed about the inheritance, rehearsing theories and counter-theories as to who might have bewitched him. Then, in an extraordinary climax, described by anthropologist W. H. Rivers, 'They utter reproaches of one village against another, and threaten fearful revenge. The wordy war leads to blows, and with cudgels and sticks to represent weapons the sorcerers fight in mockery of the combat which will follow the death of the victim'.[5] Meanwhile, a tree called by the name of the victim is felled.

Just as prayers and curses are the origins of both poetry and the doctor's prescriptions, so this play-acting is the precursor of the theatre *and* of the operating theatre.

Diagnosis and healing by tribal medicine men aim to reverse rites of bewitchment. They may begin by consulting an oracle to determine the identity of the malevolent sorcerer, and continue with counter-magic and other strategies designed to neutralize the malign influence. These can only work if the culture of the place allows them to, just as the original magic depends on the underlying cultural values which make them comprehensible to the people. The vellaymen of the South Seas remained effective as long as people could believe in their power – the opposite of the placebo effect. Such strength of belief, which is more than any one individual's faith but the collective belief of a whole society, is easily sufficient to neutralize one person's instress and bring about the failure of his life-supporting systems: the victim is simply induced by intolerable pressure in the psychic atmosphere to collapse or *implode*, like a light-bulb.

Mass collapses of instress may have been at the root of the Jonestown suicides in 1977, when 900 acolytes of the parareligious leader the 'Reverend' Jim Jones took poison at his Guyanan estate merely because he ordered them to do so. It seems to have been at the heart of the Medieval epidemics of dancing mania, which first appeared in the Rhineland during the Black Death and then – rather like the Plague itself – spread throughout northern Europe before finally dying out. This was bizarre behaviour at the very limit of comprehension, a complete loss of functional 'normality', a *socialized* catatonic frenzy. It is vividly described by the historian Barbara Tuchman.

Whether it sprang from misery or homelessness caused by heavy spring floods of the Rhine that year, or whether it was the spon-

163

taneous symptom of a disturbed time, history does not know, but the participants were in no doubt. They were convinced that they were possessed by demons. Forming circles in streets and churches, they danced for hours with leaps and screams, calling on demons by name to cease tormenting them or crying that they saw visions of Christ or the Virgin or the heavens opening. When exhausted they fell to the ground rolling and groaning as if in the grip of agonies. As mania spread to Holland and Flanders, the dancers appeared with garlands in their hair and moved from place to place like the flagellants. They were chiefly the poor – peasants, artisans, servants and beggars, with a large proportion of women, especially the unmarried.[6]

But some kind of pre-programmed cultural belief in the occult is not always the only or even necessarily the most important factor when instress spontaneously falters or fails. This is shown by the curious events of 1982 at Hollinwell, right in the heart of civilized England.

The Hollinwell incident

Sunday 13 July was a warm and pleasant day for the Hollinwell Show, an annual 'jazz festival' attended by large numbers of young, mostly female adolescents and their parents. The event has nothing to do with jazz in the usual sense; it is a competition between marching bands of young people dressed in the uniforms of chocolate soldiers. They are judged on their parade-ground skills as well as their musical ability, and the competitiveness is fierce. The following report comes from *The Times* of the next day:

> As the Warsop Marketeers juvenile jazz band was parading, the uniformed children began to stagger and collapse. Then the spectators, adults and children, also started collapsing.
> 'Some of the children were catching their friends as they fell, and were falling down themselves. No one could understand what was happening. It looked just like a battlefield, with sprawled bodies everywhere,' said Mrs Christine Williams, a bystander.

As the victims were ferried to hospital, worried Environmental Health Officers were totting up symptoms: nausea, vomiting, abdominal pain, burning eyes and a metallic taste in the mouth. It looked like a poison – perhaps some crop-spray chemical in the grass had been disturbed by the children's marching feet? Or maybe (even more worrying) there had been some leak of poison gas from a local chemical plant? There had been no communal eating that day, so food poisoning was definitely not a possibility.

Two hours after the first spate of illness, several victims were still unconscious. Others became ill whilst accompanying sick or unconscious relatives in ambulances. In all, 200 people had first aid at the show site and a further 300 received hospital treatment. Just seven were detained overnight, although symptoms recurred in some children after being sent home and several of these had to be re-admitted. On the Wednesday – three days later – a thirteen-year-old girl and both her parents, all three of whom had been free of illness at the show, collapsed and needed hospital treatment.

The medical enquiry into Hollinwell concentrated on the poisoning hypothesis. No virus could have acted so quickly, while the only other plausible explanation – mass hysteria – was regarded as a diagnosis of last resort. The crop-spray theory had to be discarded first, since no such recent activity could be discovered. The second theory – the chemical works – took a little longer to check, but officials could find no basis for it since the only possible plant was seven miles away, the wind on the day had not been in the right direction and residents in between had not been affected. So when the official report was published on 26 June it plumped unhappily for mass hysteria. Predictably the victims were angry and condemned it as a cover-up. As I have already noted, hysteria is an extremely unpopular explanation for everybody concerned.

Mass hysteria

I should immediately underline that 'mass hysteria' is distinct from the 'hysteria' discussed in the last chapter. As Brian Inglis has pointed out,[7] we are not dealing with a private neurotic condition tailored to the unique psychological requirements of the patient. Mass hysteria is a form of *group pathology* which spreads through social groups. The speed of spread varies, and the means is unknown.

Yet there is absolutely no doubt that such group pathologies existand are particularly common in certain well-defined and frequently described circumstances. Hollinwell was, in fact, a classic example of these: a concentration of young females on a warm day, marching and blowing musical instruments (i.e. potentially overbreathing) in an emotionally charged atmosphere. These circumstances occur usually in schools and, more famously, in pop concerts – especially during the world-wide epidemic of Beatlemania in the 1960s. Marching majorettes and cheerleaders are a favourite feature of American high school life and episodes similar to Hollinwell have frequently been reported from there, as they have also in Britain.

What appears to happen is that the individuals in a group suddenly begin to behave involuntarily and collectively like a single organism, as if there were automatic communication between them. Thus if one or two of them should overbreathe and faint – a temporary but sudden failure of instress – this can trigger an identical reaction right through the group. The collapse may, however, appear more serious, resembling the shock (lowering of instress) which follows traumatic injury, or even anaphylaxis – the crisis of breathlessness, urticaria and weakness which can affect severely allergic individuals after, for example, a bee-sting. Finally – and very significantly – the symptoms spread most easily from person to person along lines of emotional attachment or friendship, in the same way as the spread of earthquake damage is determined by pre-existing fault-lines in the ground. The connection with individual hysteria is the *emotional* element. Looking at old film of teenagers at pop concerts in the sixties, the most noticeable detail is that most of them are crying and screaming uncontrollably – almost competitively. In even more extreme cases, the context is often a football game or some other contest.

What are the channels which communicate this collapse of instress? I shall avoid frankly paranormal theories and mention just two hypotheses which have been advanced. The first of them is not now controversial to science, though the second is regarded as a rank heresy.

Social chemistry

Pheromones are chemicals produced in insect and animal bodies. Like hormones, our pheromones come from specialized glands and have the task of triggering remote effects. The difference is that this remoteness is very much *more* remote: pheromones do not operate on some distant organ or gland within the same body, but on the body of a completely different individual. So, instead of being released into the bloodstream, they are introduced into the outside environment via the media of our secretions – that is, in urine and sweat. Floating in the air, they then make contact with their targets through the sense of smell.

It is known that pheromones – again like hormones – have a powerful effect on the reproductive process. They provide information to other members of a species about the individual's hormonal status and readiness to mate. In humans this carries over into the more general process of sexual attraction, the enabling process of mating: love me, love my pheromones. The fact that underarm perspiration can be a means of saying 'I love you', or at least 'I fancy you', has interesting implications for the deodorant market (of course it can equally provide a negative message), but this is perhaps less remarkable than the astonishingly powerful effects it has on closely-knit groups.

The strange way in which female friends and women sharing rooms or living close to each other tend to develop synchronized menstrual cycles has often been observed, but how it happens has only recently been proved. At the Sonoma State Hospital in California, one of the staff had noticed how her cycles seemed to have a 'magnetic' effect on the menstruation of the other women she knew, bringing them into line with her own periods. Wondering if pheromones might be involved, they prepared an alcohol solution containing products of the woman's underarm perspiration. Then eight out of sixteen volunteer women in a quite different location, whose cycles were monitored for four months, had this solution dabbed thrice weekly on to their upper lip. Meanwhile the others – the controls – received only pure alcohol. The control group showed no change, but the rest were all found to have come closer in the timing of their periods to those of the woman whose pheromones they had unwittingly been smelling.[8]

Why this should happen is rather a mystery. At first glance it does not appear all that useful from an evolutionary point of view. In the early stages of human evolution, synchronized ovulation might easily reduce the birth rate, since it bunches a group's collective fertility into a few days each month – days on which males might be hunting or foraging. Evolution does not usually permit such restrictions unless there is some advantage the other way, which could be to do with helping to bind the community of women together. Pheromones are certainly involved in mother-baby recognition and bonding, and for animals they are used as indicators of identity, aggression levels, power structures and territorial rights. So, sexual chemistry aside, they are closely bound up with the chemistry of all the activities of living groups.

Looking for a pheromonal involvement in the Hollinwell incident throws up interesting comparisons with the synchronized period effect. Mass hysteria particularly affects girls and women, though not usually before puberty. There is also a strong association with groups who are in some way socially bonded – sharing an interest, or living or working side by side. If the California findings hold true universally, there is the interesting possibility that one person might act as a dominant influence on the biology of others in the group.

The obvious difference between synchronized menstrual cycles and something like Hollinwell is that mass hysteria can happen fast. It sweeps through a group of people like a gale, whereas the pheromonal effect on menstruation is very gradual. But this is also the difference in the nature of the systems affected: like the hysterical collapses which mimic them, traumatic or anaphylactic shock are by definition sudden, while the reproductive equipment is measured and deliberate. The tortoise and the hare respond to different stimuli according to their own natures.

Sheldrake's hypothesis

Rupert Sheldrake is a young high-flying biochemist whose book, *A New Science of Life*, has been described by *Nature* as 'the best candidate for burning there has been for many years'. In other words, this is a scientist who has dared to step outside orthodoxy and propose an entirely new, and so far speculative, principle in nature.

Sheldrake sets out to solve one of the basic problems in science, one which we have already met: that of morphogenesis. How does a molecule, a crystal, a bacterium, a mouse 'know' how to become what it is, in the shape and proportion which characterize it, and nothing else? If questioned about the morphogenesis of living things, most people would give a ready answer: chromosomes in the sperm and ovum combine to determine the form of a unique individual. Equipped with a computer program written in DNA code, the individual has all the instructions it needs to drive the cell-divisions and the differentiation of cells essential for its own correct development as a member of its species. The snag is that every cell contains the complete program, so how does a kidney cell know, for example, that it must follow only the instructions that apply to kidney cells and not to brain or skin cells? Jacob Bronowski said that 'cells specialize because they have accepted the DNA instructions to make the proteins that are appropriate to the functioning of that particular cell and no other. This is DNA in action'.[9] But this begs the question as to how on earth cells decide to 'accept' the DNA instructions. An even more basic problem is in the invariant structure of the program itself. What is the instress which keeps reproducing that distinctive double helix shape which contains the program and holds it together?

Sheldrake suggests the existence of an entirely new principle like – but not the same as – a 'force field'. This field influences matter so that it tends to repeat forms which have previously been formed. The more repetition that is achieved, the more this principle – which he calls a *morphogenetic field* – exerts its influence; it gathers power as a rolling snowball gathers girth. Eventually, deep pathways are established, morphogenetic channels along which sequences of change are grooved to form particular patterns. These then operate automatically unless and until some deviation or variation occurs.

As yet, Sheldrake cannot prove the existence of morphogenetic fields and the 'morphic resonance' which gives them their power across time and space, but he claims these effects can be shown experimentally. They have appeared, for example, in the strange story of McDougall's rats.

THE EDUCTION OF RATS

William McDougall was a Harvard scientist trying to show, against Darwin, that what is learned in life can be passed on to future generations: the inheritance of acquired characteristics as proposed by the Chevalier de Lamarck (1744–1829). In 1920, McDougall put rats to swim in a tank of water with two escape ramps: one attractively well-lit, but giving the rat a sharp electric shock; a second dark and unpromising, but delivering no shock. After noting how many attempts the rodents needed before learning to swim direct to the dark escape route, he then bred from this stock a new generation of rats and introduced the progeny into the tank.

McDougall continued this study for fifteen years, breeding in all thirty-eight generations of rats. As he had hoped, he found that the rats' performance did indeed get better and better with each succeeding generation, even when he changed his selection bias towards the stupider rats (see figure 4).

However, when McDougall compared these 'Lamarckian' rats with a control group of rodents *not* descended from trained stock, he found 'the disturbing fact that the groups of controls derived from this (untrained) stock in the years 1926, 1927, 1930 and 1932 show a diminution in the number of errors from 1927 to 1932'.[10] In other words, the rats seemed to be learning to use the unlit ramp more and more efficiently, *even if their parents had never learned to use it*. When the experiment was repeated even more thoroughly in Australia, the same result was found, with the added feature that even the very first generation of untrained rats *started* at the level of ability attained only after thirty generations by McDougall's rats several years earlier. The experiment knocked the Lamarckian thesis on the head, since rats from both trained and untrained stock learned at the same rate. But it opens the question: is this improving level of skill *communicated* from generation to generation and, if so, how? On Sheldrake's theory the rats learned faster because a channel of learning had been grooved by their predecessors. The existence of such a field, invisibly pushing and shaping events is by his

170

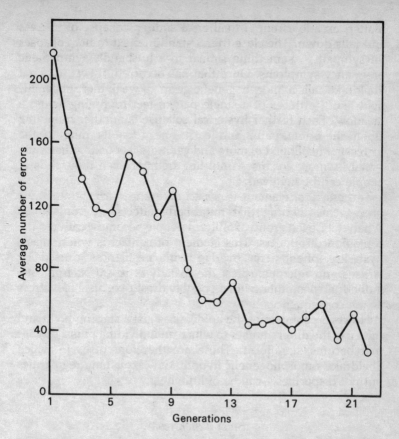

Fig. 4. *The average number of errors in successive generations of rats selected in each generation for slowness of learning. (Data from McDougall, 1938).*

own admission entirely speculative. Nevertheless, it covers the facts.

If the Sheldrake effect is at work in human learning, it must apply also to human behaviour – the patterned movement of living things generated by a combination of inheritance and learning. It would therefore be clearly at work in dancing mania or in events like the Hollinwell incident which, when they happen at different times and in diverse places, appear unique yet share many features in common.

The suggestion then is that, for reasons which may not even

matter, an adolescent girl suffers a sudden collapse of instress and falls down. The close friend standing next to her collapses 'in sympathy', something similar to a husband's sympathetic pregnancy symptoms. Once that has occurred, it sets up what Sheldrake calls a 'morphogenetic germ', a weak morphogenetic field like the traces of a single pair of feet trampling across a meadow. Each further hysterical collapse is another trampling along the same path, and each one adds its mite to the increasing likelihood of more and yet more feet taking that route – that is, more collapses until hundreds or even thousands of people can be involved.

The essential element is *contact*. We know from the simple process of yawning that mind-body effects are contagious. When the closed group of afflicted people becomes scattered the contagion disappears. This element of contact is where mass-hysterical phenomena overlap with pestilences caused by viruses and microparasites: the malady is *passed on* from one individual to another, with a possibly drastic collapse of instress as the consequence.

However, sometimes the epidemic is just a starting point and then it is the different uses to which an individual puts a disease that become significant. These are therefore cases in which Sheldrake's morphogenetic hypothesis – explaining regularities but not disparities – can be of little help.

Sleepy sickness

Many people know of the catastrophic influenza outbreak which burned through the world in the immediate aftermath of the First World War, killing twenty-five million people. Perhaps because of the prominence of the flu, we have forgotten another even more sinister disease at work amongst the population in those days. It started in Vienna in the middle of the war and in the next twelve years attacked millions world-wide. Then in 1927 it vanished as suddenly as it had appeared, leaving almost 5 million people dead and millions more – though they did not always realize it – terribly damaged.

The first symptoms were flu-like – high fever, aching limbs and prostration. This weakness emerged in the character of an intense drowsiness, as the patient gradually slipped into a semiconscious or unconscious state with partial loss of muscle tone. In a third of such cases, death came before awakening. Some other patients, however, showed a number of contradictory neurological symptoms: sudden attacks of restlessness climaxing in bouts of wild, maniacal activity; jerks, spasms, bodily contortions; and the signs of Parkinson's disease. These were prefactory or additional to continued periods of the lethargy. Of those who recovered, many seemed able to lead nearly 'normal' lives, but for most there was a tragic and lifelong aftermath to the disease. Once they had recovered from the acute stage of illness, and for a few years thereafter, patients often experienced periodic extraordinary crises in the form of outbursts of mania and paranoia, sudden tics and compulsions, sharp episodes of horror or ecstasy. But for a great many patients a state of torpor and semi-sleep supervened; their bodies *and their minds* became frozen. In this state, abandoned in institutions, isolated and completely misunderstood, hundreds of thousands of them died. A few lived on until the coming of a drug, L-Dopa, which was able to bring them back after fifty years of this entrancement to something like normal consciousness, although in many cases the return was only temporary. Some of the patients 'awoke' with no sense that five decades had passed.[11]

Yet this picture hardly does justice to the bewildering variety of this sickness, so diverse that many of its victims, though apparently normal, lived out their remaining years driven – or intolerably burdened – by psychotic, schizophrenic or neurotic traits whose origins were unrecognized.

History may even have paid a more terrible price than we know for the pandemic. It had first appeared in Austria; just at the same time a twenty-six-year-old private soldier, under treatment for a minor wound at an army hospital near Berlin, began to formulate a systematic anti-semitism which characterized the Jews as a 'pestilence' requiring 'extermination'. The development of Hitler's bizarre personality and medical history from this time strongly suggest that he was a victim of post-encephalitic illness.[11]

Encephalitis lethargica was thought to be something new at the time of its latest appearance, yet it had been around for at least 2,000 years. As Sacks notes, it has reappeared at intervals perhaps once or twice in a century, though never apparently as virulently as in this instance. It seems to be one of a class of diseases which we have the strange capacity to forget, and which we are then painfully forced to rediscover upon each of its renewals. What causes it? A virus, presumably, capable of damaging the part of the brain involved in producing neurotransmitters, particularly the one called dopamine. This is among the body's key chemicals, whose excess seems to cause schizophrenia and whose deficiency certainly results in Parkinson's disease. In its acute phase sleepy sickness obviously lowers instress, as hundreds of diseases do, but its neurological and psychological long-term consequences are highly extraordinary. At least five hundred different disturbances of movement, mood and consciousness have been listed[13] yet there are no physical brain changes which can account for them. Sacks argues with conviction that there must be 'many other determinants of clinical state and behaviour besides localized changes in the brain.' Among these, he regards the kind of human contact available, the emotions and personality of the patient as perhaps the most important: 'the "*quality*" of the individual – his "strengths" and "weaknesses", resistances and pliances, motives and experiences, etc. played a large part in determining the severity, course and form of his illness'.[14] Later he calls the whole agonized post-encephalitic phase 'a coming-to-terms of the sensitized individual with his total environment'.

Another example of epidemic instress-failure is just as mysterious, and is particularly interesting because it has frequently been attributed to entirely psychosomatic causes. What to call it – even whether it exists at all – is still a matter of debate by distinguished medical authorities. One name for it in the medical journals is Epidemic Neuromyasthenia. It is easier to call it after the hospital where its most famous outbreak occurred.

Royal Free disease

It happened in 1955, at the height of the last great wave of polio epidemics. This was not, of course, a coincidence.

The virus for poliomyelitis is common in the environment, but it is generally less severe if contracted (usually through contamination with faeces) in the earliest years. Infection – or since 1954, vaccination – confers lifelong immunity. However, the more sterile a baby's early environment the greater its chance of avoiding infection until later in childhood, or perhaps as a young adult, when there is a greater chance of suffering the notorious consequences of the disease: devastating failure of the motor-nerve cells in the spinal cord, paralysis and perhaps death. This is the reason why, before a vaccine appeared, polio seemed to favour the more affluent classes – those, ironically, who were best educated in the germ theory and who sought to ensure protection by diligent avoidance of dirt and pollution. It was not a disease of the dirty, but of the clean.[15]

Fear of polio during the fifties was rampant, whipped to a crescendo by the polio charities' fund-raising campaigns. It was this climate in which, in a few places, polio outbreaks were shadowed by a strange and unfamiliar travelling companion – a disease whose cruel mimicry of the polio symptoms could be accounted for by no virus or apparent physical cause.

In October 1948 there was a polio case in a coastal town in Iceland. Soon, numbers of people there and in two neighbouring towns started collapsing. Medically they were found to have local muscle weakness, tenderness (but not wasting) in the limbs, an inability to concentrate and general fatigue and debility. There was no significant fever, no gross nerve damage and no deaths. However, by the next April when the epidemic abated, as many as 7 per cent of the population in these towns had been affected; and when they were followed up in 1955, only a quarter of them had fully shaken off the effects of the 'mystery illness'.

1955 was also the year of the much-debated Royal Free outbreak, which started on 13 July and ran its course until almost the end of November. By that time 292 members of the staff – 255 of whom had to be admitted as patients – were affected, the great majority of them nurses. Only a tiny number of patients were afflicted, and very few men. Symptoms were similar to the Icelandic cases, but events at the Royal Free resembled even more closely an outbreak which had occurred as long ago as 1934 at the Los Angeles County General Hospital, when 198 medical staff (4.5 per cent of the total) went down with "systemic and meningeal symptoms resembling polio".[16] Los Angeles was undergoing a polio epidemic at the time.

Events at the Royal Free also resembled the much smaller epidemic two years earlier at London's Middlesex Hospital, where during a period of two and a half months fourteen nurses had gone down with a variety of symptoms, none identical in any patient but all having some resemblance to an aspect of polio. Writing about the Middlesex outbreak almost thirty years later, two doctors who were there had come to doubt that there was any single disease: "We think that the fourteen patients became a homogenous group only after admission, and that the symptoms then produced were due to a preoccupation with poliomyelitis on the part of doctors and patients.'[17]

There was no coincidental polio outbreak at the Royal Free in 1955, but polio was still very much in the air owing to the publicity around the vaccine's discovery in the previous year. When nurses and other hospital staff began to go sick with half the signs of polio, every effort was made to find a pathogenic organism capable of causing the illness. In spite of all the resources of one of London's great teaching hospitals, no such organism could be found, and the official medical enquiry had to content itself with an explanation of 'no explanation'. Later suggestions attributing the outbreak to mass hysteria have always been passionately rebutted, but *dis*passionately this does seem the most likely explanation.

What is interesting to me is the contrast between Hollinwell and the Royal Free. The closed-group hysteria of Beatlemania – to which more obviously 'medical' incidents like Hollinwell are related – is sudden, coming on like a flash-flood. Once the symptoms are gone, the victims probably feel no long-term after-effects. However, after the Los Angeles General epidemic of para-polio, more than half of the victims were still off work *six months later*. When twenty-one of them were re-examined between fourteen and eighteen *years* later, all still had some slight movement disorders. Victims of the Royal Free had similar apparently permanent effects and as a result of their long-term disabilities, they deeply resent the hysteria label.

However, whatever the 'formal' cause of any illness, it belongs to the person who suffers it. To call them patients, then, may be entirely correct; on the other hand, there will be occasions when to call them 'victims' may be entirely inappropriate.

Electing to die

I started this chapter by asking 'Why do we stay alive?' The answer that most satisfies me is that we decide to do so. The body is made up of living cells and each has a kind of life of its own, partaking in the life of all the others. Each cell influences and is influenced by the connections and communications which continually maintain life – the condition which I have referred to as instress. Instress is not something you set up and then walk away from; it has to be held in place, and the decision to continue to do that is made in every waking and sleeping moment of our lives, at every level of our being.

The human organism knows how to develop from a single fertilized cell into the 100,000,000,000,000 cells of the grown person. It knows how to create the patterns, interconnections, symmetries and transformations which maintain that vast structure. It *knows* how to live and also that life must be chosen. Seven out of every ten fertilized embryos fail to make that choice. It is impossible to say how many people – having once embarked on life – nevertheless choose to opt out. Clearly if harmless skin diseases can be produced at will, instress too can be destroyed – consciously or otherwise – and lead to death.

We know, for instance, that recently bereaved people have a much higher death rate than the rest of us. The loss of a significant relationship and subsequent failure to find a substitute is one of the cancer risk-factors we have considered. We have also seen the widowers' doubled death rate from coronary heart disease. Mourning is itself both a necessary but, if inappropriately prolonged, a quite dangerous activity, as is recognized in Chapter 38 of the *Book of Ecclesiasticus* with its advice to the bereaved:

'Weep bitterly and make great moan, and use lamentation as he is worthy, and that a day or two, lest thou be evil spoken of: and then comfort thyself for thy heaviness. For of heaviness cometh death, and the heaviness of the heart breaketh strength.'

There is even evidence that the *mode* of death can be 'chosen'. Dr Ben Fletcher, a psychologist at Hatfield Polytechnic, was doing some work on the links between men's occupations and their causes of death. He found definite correlations, some of them not particularly predictable: that soldiers and accountants share a predilection for death by cancer, and that policemen and telephonists run a significantly higher-than-normal risk of heart disease. These results are interesting in themselves, but there is something more. Fletcher compared the men's causes of death with those of their wives, hoping to highlight further the links between diseases and specific occupations. Instead he stumbled on something very much more remarkable. Working on deaths which occurred in Britain during the sixties and seventies, he showed that wives – whatever their occupation – have *almost the same disease risk-profile as their husbands*. The wife of a policeman shares more than just hearth and police home with her husband, she shares a similar high risk of circulatory disease; likewise a soldier's and an accountant's wife of death by cancer; and so on through every occupation on his list.

These are statistical results achieved by averaging the figures from more than a million deaths and as such, they need to be used with a degree of care. But they are highly suggestive of the way in which the mind-bodies of emotionally close people function in tandem. Given the facts already noted earlier about such things as synchronized menstruation and mind-caused epidemics, it is perhaps not very surprising that when it comes to the self-removal of instress through disease, we are not quite so individual as we think.

We live in time and are creatures of it. But we are also in our very essence *users* of it. The timings of life, the rhythms and chronicities, are vital to us and we hang our personalities on them. So, too, can we time death. When the American sociologist David Phillips was researching his doctoral thesis on 'Dying as a form of social behaviour'[18] he stumbled across a peculiar dip in the death rate of practising Jews immediately before the major Jewish festival of Yom Kippur, or Day of Atonement. There was no equivalent drop in the general population's death rate at this time. To understand why this might happen – and Phillips found it not only in New York, but also among the Jews of Budapest – we need to appreciate that Yom Kippur is an occasion of unrivalled emotional importance in the Jewish calendar. Its observance is above all a *family* obligation with all the emotional force which that implies, including the tradition of paying a visit to the graves of close relatives. It was as if Jews were so reluctant to miss the festival that they were capable, to a significant extent, of *postponing death until it was over*. Phillips wondered if the same effect could be observed in other emotionally important cyclic occasions, so he looked at birthdays. Sure enough, he found that we are statistically less likely to die just before our birthdays than at other times, and statistically *more* likely to do so just afterwards.

But if death can be staved off in this way, can it also be invited with the same degree of accuracy? My own grandfather, at the age of only sixty-three and going into hospital for a minor routine operation, had a premonition of death. He made his will and other necessary arrangements, unknown to his wife and eight children. They would no doubt have been very surprised, but also mildly amused at what most people would regard as unnecessary apprehension. It is quite possible that his actions were motivated by anxiety combined with pessimism, although it would have been quite out of character: the son of a hypochondriac, he was himself not at all hypochondriacal. If that is not the explanation, then he must have had a genuine 'warning'. But where would such a premonition come from? Was it 'ordinary' extra-sensory perception? Or had he, somewhere in his unconscious, simply made the decision to die and was now informing himself of that decision? At all events, election or coincidence, he did in fact die without regaining consciousness from the anaesthetic.

A much more clear-cut case of someone making an appointment with death is quoted by Gordon Rattray Taylor, which I give in his own words:

A doctor named Arnold Cowan wrote to a British medical journal to report that a patient of his suffering from cancer told him on Tuesday that he should not make his usual Thursday visit to see him, as he would be dying at 2.30 the following afternoon. He learned later that his patient had summoned the members of his family to say farewell after lunch on the Wednesday. His wife being detained for a few moments, he sent a message for her to hurry so that she would not miss the event. At 2.30 precisely, he sighed, raised both his hands above his head, smiled, and passed away.[19]

In this chapter I have tried to show that collapse or failure of the body, in some or all of its systems can be a *mental* phenomenon independent of – or perhaps working alongside – any organic pathology. Such collapses – the bursting of the cells' bubbles – I have called a failure of instress, and this is particularly susceptible to the influence of other individuals. In the next chapter, we must consider the equally powerful interpersonal influence which operates between doctor and patient.

============ *Chapter 9* ============

Patients and pleasing

**'He that is not free is not an Agent but a
Patient'**
John Wesley

*A*ll social insects and animals behave more or less hierarchic-
ally. Whether for lions or lemurs or the Labour Party, there are
protocols of deference built into nature itself. Of course
humans, being uniquely rational and cultural animals, have got
further beyond the extreme enslavement of the termite's nest
than other social creatures. The degree of our freedom, which
comes from the consciousness of choice and the will to exercise
consent, is in fact the yardstick of our humanity. Yet we are
far from having entirely escaped the termite's inheritance. The
tendency to institute pecking orders and chains of command
underlies all our societies and, though normally balanced by the
individualizing impulse, the desire to dictate and bow down, to
drive and be driven, does occasionally well up and smash down
our libertarian conceptions with overwhelming emotional force.

When there is danger, the appreciation of freedom and the
normal self-preservation instincts of 'the selfish gene' can be
temporarily suspended. Then we revert to corporate beings,
unable to act or choose as individuals do. The *emotional*
component of this is important; such abnegations are
accompanied by very strong feelings, a hint that these may be
part of an atavistic trait.

When such a trait comes into effect the result may be cringing,
crawling servility or else the very heights of heroic selflessness.
Totalitarianism knows and exploits this – the rise of Nazism
happened because of it and it made possible the Gulag Archi-
pelago and the Jonestown suicides. But nobler examples also
come to mind. The dance musicians of the *Titanic* steadfastly

playing ragtime as the ship dipped below the glacial sea; the Spartans at Thermopylae, combing each other's hair; the tiny fragment of a Welsh regiment which faced the entire nation of Zulu warriors at Rorke's Drift and sang 'Men of Harlech'. People in such plight – as Wesley says – have stopped being agents and become patients.

The same route is taken by someone who becomes a medical patient. First an individual is healthy and free. Then sickness threatens. After a time, if the sick person despairs of a self-made remedy, he places himself in the hands of another authority; then he ceases to be an agent and becomes a patient. Becoming a patient is – as Jonathan Miller says – a transition into a new way of being, consciously chosen:

> . . . you change your social identity, turning yourself from someone who helps himself into someone who accepts the orders, routine and advice of qualified experts. You submit to the rules and recommendations of a profession, just as a novice submits to the rules and recommendations of his or her chosen order.[1]

Equally postulant-like, you have 'for your own good' abdicated your freedom.

In 1623, the poet and priest John Donne wrote his *Devotions Upon Emergent Occasions*. These were prompted by his own severe illness and, in spite of the writer's devotional intent, the book attains particular greatness as one of the most acute accounts ever written of the experience of being a patient *in extremis*. Donne says: 'I cannot rise out of my bed till the physician enable me, nay I cannot tell that I am able to rise till he tell me so. I do nothing, I know nothing of myself: how impotent a piece of the world is any man alone! And how much less a piece of *himself* is that man!'[2]

Some patients do not achieve patience. They become furious at the impotence described by Donne, particularly when they look back at the acute phase of their illness when they were no longer able to maintain normal dignity or the accustomed liberty of thought (let alone action) which as human beings they value above all else.[3] Perhaps every patient feels this to some extent: shame and disgust at the abjectness of the sick. But Donne, though he chafes, knows it is best to be philosophic. He has already stressed in his famous phrase that 'No man is an island'

and, though he knows the doctor-patient relationship to be an unequal and rather artificial one, nevertheless human contact is a prerequisite of recovery and, to the lonely and easily-shunned patient, this is the best contact available.

Of course, there really is good reason for surrendering to another authority under threat of illness. The sick often flourish by losing themselves in the medical (or nursing) process. The doctor (or nurse) seems eager to take responsibility, extending a curing absolution to the patient – and this really can cure. It is part of a general adaptive survival mechanism which operates in every human culture, however primitive or advanced. Authoritative – even authoritarian – healers are needed everywhere.

Placebo

The sick person becomes a patient by abandoning self-assertiveness and seeking help 'under' a doctor. But even though the doctor is imbued with confidence, the disease may be beyond the reach of clinical skill. Vigorous measures may be taken, yet these could be useless or even potentially harmful. In this case, objectively speaking, the doctor has nothing to offer except energy, optimism and buoyancy, yet these may be all that are needed for healing to occur. It is called the *placebo effect*.

Placebo might lay claim to be one of the most important principles in the whole of medicine and it is thought to have some influence on two out of three doctor-patient encounters. In one out of three, the effect is marked. Interestingly, this closely parallels a widely accepted estimate of the incidence of successful hypnosis.

Placebo is respected by medical science, but largely for its nuisance value. It interferes with the objective business of drug evaluation, since you cannot always tell whether a response is 'real' or placebo. Thus complicated protocols have to be followed in clinical trials, whereby patients are divided into two groups – one group receiving the active medication while the other has, say, chalk pills or a saline injection. It is important that the medical staff administering the therapy is also ignorant of which group is which, since it is known that the attitude of the doctor or nurse has an important effect; it is as if their expectation communicates itself to the patient, even though no one says a word. A third level of control comes in when the *evaluator* of the treatment is also ignorant of the distribution of patients between the groups (the *triple-blind* trial), for subjectivity can skew the picture here too.

The word translates from Latin as 'I shall please'. *Placebo Domino*, meaning 'I'll please the Lord', is a phrase from the Catholic rite of Vespers of the Dead, and in common English was used to refer to any servile person. Its use in medicine started before doctors had acquired a high social standing, at a time when they too were fairly servile and would commonly prescribe salt or chalk pills just to satisfy the patient's expectations and earn their fee. These inert medicines often had a surprising effect; the patient's faith in them seemed capable of lowering a fever or reducing a swelling in a remarkable way. If the *doctor* had faith, too, the response might be doubled! Until the middle of this century most medicine achieved its success in this way.

The placebo is not entirely a matter of the doctor trying to please *the patient*. As we have seen, when the patient is *in extremis* the boot is on the other foot. Now the doctor has the whip hand and the pleasing must flow, if at all, in the other direction, with the patient deferring to the doctor. Donne ably describes the patient's anxiety about the doctor's frame of mind: 'I observe the Physician with the same diligence as he the disease; I see he fears, and I fear with him.' Yet the doctor tries to hide his fear: 'He knows that his fear shall not disorder the practice and exercise of his Art, but he knows that my fear may disorder the effect and working of his practice.' This is as true as ever it was and it means that, even in the modern clinical setting, the patient and doctor engage in a complicated game of reciprocal bluffing. The patient craves reassurance from the doctor and, receiving it, is helped to heal. But how is the doctor to be reassuring? Of course he or she may be a very good actor, but confidence is the main ingredient – a confidence that communicates itself. This confidence will be redoubled if, in the course of treatment, the patient is found to be responding. So if the patient can 'please the doctor' – which most 'good' patients try to do anyway – this may result in a beneficial feedback. (Note that this implies a more sinister side of placebo – the 'nocebo' response, in which any negative expectations on the part of medical staff may be picked up and fulfilled.)

The origin of our need for external authority to take charge in sickness or distress is two-fold. As we have seen above, it is partly the ancient instinct of self-abnegation in face of fear, but it is also a kind of reversion to infancy. Human childhood is relatively longer than that of any other animal. Obviously a lengthy period of training for our emotions and responses is necessary, because we own minds of extraordinary complexity and variety. Some of the side-effects of this have already been noted, particularly in respect of sexual conditioning. Arthur Koestler believed, more fundamentally, that the child's long period of dependence 'may be at the root of the adult's ready submission to authority, and his quasi-hypnotic susceptibility to doctrines and ethical commandments – his urge to *belong*, to identify himself with a group, or its leader, or its system of beliefs.[4] If this is right, we are not only *instinctually* inclined (under certain circumstances) to need authority; we are also conditioned to need it. The emotional charge of the primitive instinct combined with childhood training is enormous. This emotion is the power at the disposal of the placebo effect.

Pleasing and loving

The simplest application of placebo is with a young child. The toddler is quite terrifyingly resilient physically; it is very difficult to break her pliant bones, her blood clots with supreme efficiency, she hardly knows what pain is and she simply sleeps through her more debilitating fevers and infections. Psychologically, however, she is much more vulnerable. She needs above all a loving environment, and it is this that gives her such very good placebo responses. So when she falls off her trike on the stone-flagged garden path, she runs to her mother to be 'kissed better'. No parent of young children needs telling how extraordinarily effective 'kissing better' is.

Quite simply, it is love which is the active ingredient in this medicine. Not just the mother's for the child, but the child's love for the mother is what I believe eases the pain, swelling and shock. How does mere love, a nebulous and fickle enough emotion, manage to be so physically powerful? Familial love such as the child and mother share is complicated, but for convenience let us say in this case that it consists of faith, hope and charity in roughly equal parts.

First, *faith* is there because the child believes the mother cares for her and wants her to be well. Acutally, belief is necessary for all love, because all love is intrinsically a perception (however mistaken) of truth – 'my love is true, be true to me'. Next, *hope* is the child's expectation of feeling better, a measure of confidence in the power of the mother's kiss. Finally, *charity* is the ability to exclude any reservations and to give oneself over uncritically to another person's ministration. This is covered by St Paul in his famous prescription when he says that 'charity vaunteth not itself, is not puffed up, doth not behave itself unseemly, seeketh not her own, is not easily provoked, thinketh no evil'. The child at moments of crisis has a natural affinity for charity. Here again is that element of self-abnegation, so clearly tied in with our emotions.

Freud's equation of the bond between hypnotist and subject with people bound by a loving relationship was eventually extended to the bond between analyst and patient, which among other things helped him to account for transference. Does the insight apply equally outside psychoanalysis? And if so, does it account for the placebo effect? We might explore this idea by considering the conditions under which medical placebo seems to be particularly effective.

Placebo's arcadia

According to Edward Shorter, the period between the wars can be regarded as a Golden Age of placebo.[5] It is now generally agreed that until the Second World War, most medical techniques had little scientific validity and were objectively useless for the treatment of serious illness. But of course that is not how medicine presented itself at the time. Doctors took much of the credit for the noticeably elongated and more healthy life-expectancy of the first decades of the century, though these were actually to do with rising living standards and better drains. The misplaced laurels did, however, serve to build up an impressive store of public faith and support for medicine. While the objective skill of the doctor was yet small, his subjective credit – by contrast with earlier and also more recent times

– was great. These indeed look like ideal conditions for placebo, but the general feeling that medicine was 'going somewhere' and 'finding the answers' is not quite enough; so, taking the child being kissed better as the model placebo-responder, we might look a little deeper into the doctor-patient relationship during that Golden Age between the wars.

For example, how much *faith* did patients have that medicine really *cared* about them? This was before the National Health Service, when you paid for your medical care – implying, perhaps, a commercial rather than a caring relationship. But apparently the two were not mutually exclusive. Shorter says that in the 1920s there would be an average of three and a half house-calls per illness, and two and a half for cases of the common *cold*! In fact, doctors were expected to call on a sick patient at least every day. On the other hand, if a patient came to them, they spent much longer in the consulting room than they would today. Most patients who consulted regularly suffered then as now from various psychogenic illnesses, and the doctors' recognition of their own impotence forced them to rely on sympathy, and on giving patients the chance to talk through their symptoms.

As to hospital medicine, we must not forget the importance of nursing. After mangling both legs in a flying accident in 1931, the fighter pilot Douglas Bader lay for weeks in a Reading hospital, hanging on to life as if by a spider's web. He always maintained later that he owed his survival to Nurse Dorothy Brace's dedicated round-the-clock attention: 'Twenty-two hours, give or take an hour, of every tenuous day, seven days a week,' says one of Bader's biographers.[6] In many ways nursing is an even more fundamental part of healing then doctoring, since its whole basis is care and attentiveness.

The next element in our ideal loving realationship is *hope*. What governs the patient's confidence in clinical effectiveness is context and the physician's bearing. We have seen that in the twenties and thirties medicine, though increasingly good at diagnosis, was fairly impoverished in terms of effective treatment. It was the doctors' and nurses' unhesitating and undoubtedly sincere confidence which maintained their prestige.

Often the more elaborate and drastic a treatment, the more confidence a patient can invest in it. Certainly, one of the oldest rules for placebo treatment is that a nasty-tasting medicine is twice as good as a palatable one. In the fifties, when the medical profession's credit was still very high, a not unusual treatment for *angina pectoris* – which even now is difficult to control – was to open the chest and tie the mammary artery. This was reported as bringing relief in up to 75 per cent of cases, supposedly by altering the area's blood flow. Eventually, the procedure was tested against a sham operation to see if it was any better than placebo. It is unusual to see placebo-controlled trials of surgery, so the results of this one are of particular interest. It turned out that of the (unknowing) placebo patients, who under anaesthetic and the full panoply of the operating theatre merely had their skin incised and then sewn up again, 43 per cent experienced both subjective and objectively assessed improvement. Of those who really had their mammary arteries tied, only 32 per cent improved![7]

Hope and expectation are entirely mental matters, of course, but they can have dramatic effects on the way our body feels. Pavlov gave a partial answer to how this works in his investigation of conditioning, and his Soviet successors have continued the work. In one experiment[8] patients suffering from urinary fistulas were fitted with gauges to show the pressure of the urine in their bladders. At first their subjective (and accurate) feeling of a full bladder coincided with the reading of 'FULL' on the meter. But, unknown to the patients, the psychologists fiddled the gauges to make them work in reverse, so that now 'FULL' meant 'empty' and vice versa. Completely bamboozled, the patients began to find their bodies trusting to the hospital hardware more than their own sensations. Thus when the gauge showed 'FULL' they would have an uncontrollable urge to urinate – even though their bladders were in fact virtually empty. If it showed 'EMPTY', they felt no such urge although their bladders would actually be almost full.

This is possibly the kind of experiment which can only be done in the USSR. Certainly if patients anywhere began to suspect that this kind of thing was being done on any sort of scale, the prospects for continued placebo would be bleak! Perhaps this is the problem today, at least in part. If patients think medicine is too 'scientific', while they possibly appreciate the gain in knowledge if it can be applied to them, they may nevertheless worry as to whether they are patients in the traditional sense or a few strokes on the computer keyboard. At all events, it does seem that the Golden Age of medical placebo is now behind us. All three of the legs which once supported the 'loving relationship' between healer and patient are considerably less steady.

Tattered faith

Faith in the capacity of the medical professions to *care* has been severely tested in the years since the first really effective drugs began to be discovered. Shorter refers to this as the 'post-modern' period in the history of doctor-patient relationships, starting after the Second World War and coinciding in Britain with the establishment of the National Health Service. The emphasis on *successful* science brought a new thrust for quantity as opposed to quality. Centralized technical facilities and econ-omies of scale become paramount. Very large high-technology hospitals proliferated, with their impersonal long corridors, computerized nursing stations and science-fiction operating theatres; anything parochial or small-scale was, if possible, closed down. It seems obvious that a health service which drifts away from the people in this way is bound to lose allegiance.

William Carlos Williams, doctor and poet, wrote with little affection about hospitals in his *Autobiography*:

Obviously enough, the entire world today is a hospital so that, one thing cancelling another, that makes hospital a very normal environment. It is only incidentally concerned with illness: quite casually, to itself, it measures with some indifference the decay of flesh, its excreta, bad odours and even its ecstasies of birth and cure. Cure to a physician is a pure accident, to the pathologist in his laboratory almost a disappointment. The real thing is the excitement of the chase, the opportunity for the exercise of precise talents, the occasion for batting down a rival to supercede him, to strut, to boast and get on with one's fellows. Discovery is the great goal – and the accumulation of wealth.[9]

Williams was writing in the late 1940s, at which time his point cannot really have seemed all that 'obvious'. Indeed, it must have seemed an outrageous slur. Yet today – next to the thoughts of Ivan Illich and other critics of medicine – the paragraph seems emotional and perhaps harsh, but not particularly controversial. The sense in recent years has been of a profession turned away from a hostile world and inwards, absorbing itself in its own enthusiasms and problems. In America this has been compounded by a major embarrassment – the public's new-found willingness to sue doctors for malpractice. This litigation tears the profession apart and forces doctors to be insured for millions of dollars. In Britain there are different but equally wounding internecine episodes. One of these was the Savage case, where an enquiry into the East London obstetrician's competence exposed a degree of jealousy and rancour within one of the world's oldest teaching hospitals such as would not have been out of place in a small palace in Renaissance Italy.

The patient's 'post-modern' encounters with doctors are no more encouraging. The average GP consultation time in Britain is between 5 and 7 minutes per patient. Daytime house calls are fairly rare – and never every day. Night house calls are increasingly farmed out to deputizing agencies, whose 'flying-squad' doctors are robotized diagnosis-machines intent on keeping personal contact to a minimum. Meetings with hospital consultants can also be brutishly short. Dr Oliver Sacks in his account of his own illness describes how, with the 'pre-med' already inside him, he waited anxiously to speak to his surgeon:

> Mr Swan made his appearance at 8.53 and found me gazing at my watch. I had a momentary impression of a very shy man, but this was instantly effaced by his brisk, hearty voice.
> 'Well', he said loudly. 'How are we doing today?'
> 'Bearing up', I replied, and my voice sounded muzzy.
> 'Nothing to worry about,' he continued briskly. 'You've torn a tendon. We reconnect it. Restore continuity. That's all there is to it . . . nothing at all!'
> 'But . . .' I said slowly – but he had already gone from the room.[10]

This was the patient's only pre-operative discussion with the man who, in a few minutes time, would cut his leg open. I am told that it would be very unusual for a surgeon not even to examine the leg before operating: but of course it is above all the lack of *personal* communication which rankles with the patient.

Battered hope

What confidence is there in orthodox medicine's power to *cure*? In 1985 Dr David Axelrod, New York State Commissioner for Health, publicly denounced a commercial health care system which prefers profits to patients and allows malpractice (and malpractice insurance) to run out of control. In Axelrod's opinion American hospitals are wholly unsafe places, full of infection risks, medical accidents, incompetence and dangerous radiation. Even more amazing was his excoriation of doctors. 'Doctors are not the healers they think they are. The patient himself is the healer,' said the Commissioner. 'If you don't need a doctor, don't go to one and if you do, deal with them as aggressively as you would any salesman'.[11]

But Americans have already picked up the message. Trust in doctors has given away to cynicism, which in turn has yielded to an aggressive new type of patient demand. This has two almost contradictory results. Pulling in one direction, it stimulates the ever-increasing technical investment by hospitals and clinics, for in our world patients exercising choice and physicians looking for jobs are liable to opt for the most 'modern' facility. This – along with other spiralling costs such as malpractice insurance – has helped to produce extraordinary inflation in US health care. In 1950 the average unit cost (per patient per year) was $87. This rose to $137 by 1960 and to only $147 by 1970. Then came the explosion: by 1980, the figure stood at $1,000 – an annual increase *eight times greater than the rate for the whole previous decade*. (See figure 5).

A few years ago George Pickett, MD, president of the American Public Health Association, put it like this: 'In no other system does rising demand produce price-increases and supply-decreases simultaneously.' He added, ominously: 'In no other economic system does the boss make all the decisions while everyone else takes all the risks'.[12] These critics, of course, come from the beleaguered *public* health field in a country whose medical resources are largely dominated by private health. Private health insurance premiums in the US are inflating by 25 per cent a year. Many individuals are insulated from this because, as employees, they are insured in corporate schemes. This shifts concern to the employers, who see health as a

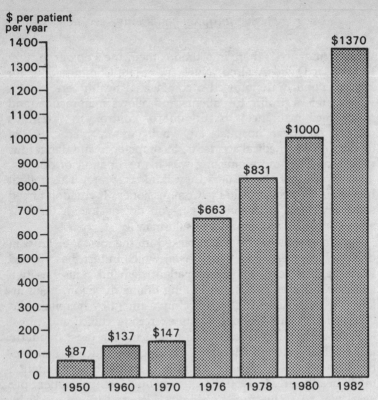

Fig. 5. *Average U.S. health costs per person per year. 1950–1982.*

looming factor on their balance sheets. Chrysler spends more on health than on steel or rubber.

Sour charity

Consumers do not surrender themselves; they stand on their rights, remaining eternally on guard and suspicious. This is just another way of saying that, without faith and hope, there *can* be no charity, no 'loving relationship' at all between healer and patient and ultimately no placebo. I am not saying that the placebo effect has disappeared from surgeries and consulting rooms. Even within the system there are bound to be individuals creating effective healing conditions, as there will be patients who respond well to 'high tech' management. But in general the outlook for healing and caring appears to be bleaker, and this has an effect on the general health picture. Far from decreasing under the assault of post-modern medicine, illness seems to be increasing. Moreover, there does not seem to be much difference between the socialized medicine of Britain and the commercialized scene in the United States. A factor common to both sides of the Atlantic is that the quasi-hypnotic state which the medical profession once maintained has now been broken: too often there is as little love as possible lost between doctor and patient. Love is too time-consuming, too exhausting, too *expensive*. But, as we have seen, it is essential.

Medicalization

The alternative proposed by both technological doctors and consumer-patients has been 'medicalization', whose influence is so extensive that it has caused fundamental experiences to be redefined. Pregnancy and birth in the busy central obstetrics department become rather like battery-chicken affairs, risk-free and centralized for better quality-control. Believers in natural childbirth fear that soon Britain will match the US 'achievement' of one in five births by caesarian section, preferred by many obstetricians because it is a 'safer' procedure than vaginal birth.

In true Newspeak style, medicalization manipulates words so that our thinking can be compressed and fitted into the new order. So now a patient becomes – in the administrator's audit – an aggregate of QALYs. Pain becomes 'pain behaviour' and then 'learned pain behaviour'. Most fundamentally of all, even the meaning of death has been revised for the Newspeak dictionary.

To satisfy the requirements of organ transplantation, the old concept of death – that a heart has stopped beating for good – will no longer do. So now we have the more convenient idea of 'brain-death', by virtue of which the transplant team may remove a donor's organs *while the heart is still beating*, a process which is however something of a well-guarded secret and about which the donor's relatives are rarely enlightened. Dr Philip Keep, medical director of the intensive care unit at the Norwich and Norfolk Hospital, told the *Guardian*: 'You have to lie to them a bit. You say "We're going to take the organs out when he is dead." They really believe that, and I've never had the courage to tell them anything different, because I'm sure that if you actually told them what was going to happen you'd get no more donors'.[13] What happens is that the donor – having been pronounced brain-dead – is wheeled into the operating theatre like any other patient, attached to the life-support system with heart still beating and blood still circulating. If by chance the heart should stop, life-saving measures are taken just as if the patient were alive. Thus the organs' removal resembles a live operation more than a 'post-mortem', right down to the need for muscle-relaxants to prevent the still-active reflexes of the subject from jolting the scalpel. According to Dr Keep, 'The nursing staff find the whole process disturbing' and 'are conscious enough of what it is they are doing not to want people to know what actually happens.' This is not surprising, since the technological hare has far oustripped the moral tortoise of human sensibility. The result is a degree of white-lying whose ethics seem inevitably questionable.

The effects of medicalization have been described by its most passionate critic, Ivan Illich, as:

> . . . the paralysis of healthy responses to suffering, impairment and death. It occurs when people accept health management designed on the engineering model, when they conspire in an attempt to produce, as if it were a commodity, something called 'better health'. This inevitably results in the managed maintenance of life on high levels of sub-lethal illness.[14]

The Bethnal Green study, where a tendency to double-think on health has already been mentioned (see p. 77) shows the characteristic effects of the process described by Illich. In this case, the medicalization of health means using doctors and hospitals to obtain exoneration from what, at a deeper level, they are capable of believing are personal and private responsibilities. A mechanical view of the world means fatalism and not having to think or act. So, if life is too miserable to contemplate, a prescription or a 'doctor's note' become ways of escape. But the escape is short-lived. The weekly librium prescription soon turns into the occasion for self-reproach and guilt.

This is similar to the bitterness felt by Oliver Sacks when as a patient, he lost his autonomy in the surgical/medical process[15]. But for him there was compensatory healing. For the out-of-work lorry driver with 'learned pain behaviour' in his back, there may be little or no prospect of healing or a *return* to autonomy. An overburdened and misdirected health service can offer him little more in compensation than a monotonous cycle of five-minute consultations and repeat prescriptions. For the long-term resident of a thirty-bed geriatric ward never designed for the likes of her, prospects seems relatively even bleaker.

Modern health-care arrangements are in theory designed to abolish ill-health, but have ended up by increasing sickness. A good part of the reason for this is the loss of trust and a consequent falling away of placebo response, a loss which is impossible to prove but which would be a logical consequence of the kind of double-think on medicalization which I have described.

There can, of course, be no return to the previous 'modern' era of medical placebo, nor should there be. Placebo medicine as it used to be practised would be insupportably patronizing today and, in any case, once innocence has blown away you do not find it caught in a nearby thorn bush. Nevertheless, people need healing services in which they can have faith and hope, and find charity. The major charge which must be levelled at official medicine now is its encouragement of the double-think which prevents this. Its patients (or rather 'health-consumers') are divided against themselves. 'Healthy', it should not be forgotten, does not mean 'ambulant' or 'able to work' or 'functionally restored'. It still means 'whole'.

Chapter 10

Alternatives

'Your facts are useful, and yet they are not my dwelling'
Walt Whitman

*F*rom the point of view of orthodox medicine, this spreading disillusion has caused a Pandora's box of medical mischief to spring its lid. It is a box full of all the different shades of paramedic, faith healer and inner-city shaman you have ever heard of, and plenty more that you never suspected. In San Francisco, world capital of the counter-culture, there exists a directory called *Common Ground: Resources for Personal Transformation*. The listings include hundreds of unorthodox healing agencies including all the familiar bone-manipulators, psychotherapists and Eastern mystics, as well as a great many more mysterious offerings such as 'Photographic Affirmation of Growth', 'Polarity Releasing Therapy' and 'Trager Psychophysical Integration and Mentastics'.

No doubt some of this really is mischief, playing on people's ever-ready gullibility. Yet most unorthodox therapies have a clear and useful role: to fill the placebo gap left by the decline of medicine's esteem. Many of these alternative practitioners are explicit about the role of caring and emotional closeness between healer and patient. 'Listening hands use gentle touch to facilitate relaxation', says one advertisement. In another a doctor is 'especially interested in working in depth with people to understand why they are experiencing illness'. Yet another 'alternative' doctor even says, 'I like to function as an old-style family GP.'

Indeed, in some parts of America it is increasingly hard to find a family doctor. One New Yorker told me that to get one in Manhattan he had resorted to persuading a medically qualified friend to act in this capacity. The friend agreed, but they both wondered how well-qualified he was for this task since he is a renowned gastro-intestinal specialist. So while he has unrivalled knowledge of epithelial disorder, he is unlikely to be better at dealing with fatigue or a headache than a good masseur or even a good grandmother!

In Britain, comprehensive family doctor provision still theoretically exists. GPs try to fulfil the ideals of family practice, although most would agree that time, pressure and the mechanization at the heart of hospital medicine work against them. There is a similar picture throughout western Europe and an explosion of alternative – or, as it sometimes prefers to be called, complementary – medicine has occurred to compensate. In this chapter I shall consider some unorthodox approaches which seem particularly relevant to the themes I have been discussing.

Homeopathy

At the end of the eighteenth century, Samuel Hahnemann invented homeopathy virtually from scratch. To begin with, he was a conscientious scientist, though hardly a conventional one even for his own day. But as he grew older Hahnemann developed increasingly into a metaphysical thinker – almost a messianic and certainly a fanatical figure.

Hahnemann's method consisted essentially in the use of drugs ('remedies') to cure illness. But whereas allopathy (see p. 19) tries to correct symptoms by counteraction, homeopathy invokes the old Hippocratic principle of 'like cures like'. Thus the homeopath prescribes only remedies which, in a healthy person, are capable of provoking the same symptoms as those of the disease under treatment. This means, for instance, that unlike most procedures of orthodox medicine, vaccination is a homeopathic procedure.

Homeopathic remedies are prepared by diluting the active ingredient several times in water or alcohol, the ratio being one to ten parts each time. In between dilutions the solution is *succussed*, or shaken for a few minutes rather as a barman shakes a cocktail, though there is never any mixture of ingredients in homeopathy. Dilutions up to as many as 300 can be made before the resulting solution is incorporated in the characteristic small spherical pills. Succussion, it should be noted, is regarded as crucial to the 'potentising' of the remedy.

Although at first it aspired to be recognized as a science, homeopathy is unlikely to gain scientific acceptance until two major problems are resolved. The first is to do with the nature of the homeopathic remedy. After the first twenty-four dilutions and succussions, the solution has passed the Avogadros Number – the point beyond which any molecules of the original chemical ingredient have entirely disappeared. So these solutions – or potencies, as they are called – of camphor, salt, arsenic or whatever it may be no longer actually contain any camphor, salt or arsenic. As has been said, it is like putting a soluble aspirin into the Atlantic and then drinking a mouthful. To explain the power of potentized remedies, some homeopaths maintain that succussion imprints the water in some way with the power of the original ingredient, but as yet no convincing explanation has been given as to how this might happen.

The second difficulty is over research. For Hahnemann's followers, even in his own lifetime, the theory of homeopathy had reached the status of unimpeachable principle, which their inventor had nailed like Luther's 95 theses to the allopathic doors. Anyone questioning these doctrines from within the embattled ranks of the faithful was soon denounced as a heretic. So, although thousands of drugs were 'proved' to find out what symptoms they provoked – and therefore what diseases they antagonized – there was never any tradition of systematically testing the effectiveness of homeopathic drugs against the diseases themselves.

However, if it is a doubtful starter in the scientific rat-run, homeopathy has an undeniable claim as one of the healing arts. The very fact that it is unwilling to conduct large-scale trials is here much in its favour, since trials necessarily treat patients as counters and diseases as if they were objective quantities. In fact, one of the reasons why homeopaths oppose research is that the objectification of disease is against their most fundamental principles.

My own experience seems not untypical. Trying for the umpteenth time to be rid of my psoriasis, I attended London's long-established Nature Cure Clinic, where homeopathy is practised by medically qualified staff. The first time he met me, the doctor spent forty-five minutes sizing me up. That is a much more accurate phrase than 'taking the history', for it was far more thorough and wide-ranging than any such conventional procedure. It was a raw November day and I remember that at one point, a shade aggressively, he threw open the window. By observing my reaction, he wanted to know whether I had a 'warm' or a 'cold' constitution. He questioned me about my habits, hobbies and preferences. He wanted to know about my sex life and my tastes in food, what stressed and what relaxed me. Ultimately, for my skin at any rate, the treatment was not successful; but as an exercise in relating to the 'whole patient', this first consultation could not be faulted.

The emphasis on the personal nature of disease – giving patients a sense of their own high worth – gave homeopathy a useful lead in the placebo stakes right from the start. If placebo is, as I have argued, enhanced by the interpersonal quality of treatment, then Hahnemann was bound to triumph over the allopathy of his time, which relied to an insane extent on such barbarisms as repeated blood-letting and the use of poisonous 'specifics' in huge doses. The general superiority of homeopathy at that time seems to have been demonstrated particularly in the cholera pandemic of the 1830s. The illness was new to Europe and its virulence caused widespread panic, among doctors no less than in the general population. Hahnemann apparently did not panic, for he was sure of his method. On first hearing of the outbreak of the disease, he asked for a detailed report of the symptoms and on this report alone he based a homeopathic regime, whose most important element was camphor in a saturated (not a diluted or potentized) solution. Survival for cholera victims treated homeopathically was everywhere more likely than for allopathy. In orthodox hospitals, more than half the victims were dying. Of those treated with Hahnemann's regime, deaths were never more than one-third. In the Homeopathic Hospital in Golden Square, London, only one-sixth of the cholera patients succumbed as compared with an average of 53.2 per cent in the orthodox hospitals. Once the epidemic was over, reports of the relative success of homeopathy proved so embarrassing to the General Board of Health – precursor of the British government's Department of Health – that it attempted to suppress them.

Homeopathy normally requires a lengthy consultation in order to locate the individual origin of the illness, and it is therefore surprising to find it so effective in the case of a lightning infection like cholera which can kill in a matter of hours. If this suggests an objective basis for the 'like cures like' idea – a suggestion which has been strengthened by a recent successful trial of homeopathy with hay fever patients in Glasgow[1] – it does not for me quite remove the suspicion that homeopathy is above all, and in the right hands, a particularly effective and useful harnessing of the placebo effect.

The mystique of the homeopathic doctrine, the appeal to the authority of Hahnemann and the early provers of remedies, the subjective view of illness and the interpersonal almost confessional nature of the consultation all support the impression that homeopathy has more of a religious than a scientific slant. As such, it can perform a psychological martialling of the patient's own healing resources as scientific medicine can no longer do to the same extent, while having virtually no possible harmful effects. This, as I hope I have made clear, is not cause to dismiss it.

Hypnosis

I suggested in the last chapter that placebo effect is a function of the psychological process of becoming a patient, and submitting to an authoritative (even authoritarian) healer. Hypnotherapy is the most dramatic example of pure authoritarian healing I can think of, when the patient knowingly submits to a deliberate therapeutic hijack of his mind. Under hypnosis his will and beliefs can be manipulated by the therapist in such a way, it is hoped, as to activate intrinsic healing processes.

Ever since Anton Mesmer began to use trance-states systematically to cure people in the eighteenth century, the objective existence of these states has been doubted by scientists and enthusiasts of 'common sense' alike. How can a person be induced to surrender consciousness and yet act, under direction, like a conscious person? Worse, how in this state can someone be made to do anomalous things or adopt alien character traits? These effects are not 'real', surely, but play-acting? Even more mysterious is *post-hypnotic suggestion*, where the patient can be directed while in a trance to behave in certain ways *once the trance is over*. Thus a hypnotized subject may be told that after he has been 'woken up', he will scratch his head whenever he hears the word 'plum'. This he will faithfully do quite unconsciously until re-hypnotized, although the suggestion may in time wear off naturally.

Mesmer, the Austrian peasant's son whose achievements made him rich and a celebrity across Europe, evolved a theory of his own to explain these trance states. They came, he thought, from the generation of 'animal magnetism', an extrapolation from the magnestism of metals mixed with some leftover aspects of the animal spirits which had once been believed to flow through the nervous system. The mesmerist's skill was to make that magnetism flow into the subject, enhancing healing and other energetic effects.

This theory was discredited when a French Royal Commission (on which sat Benjamin Franklin, Antoine Lavoisier and the inventor of the guillotine) found that biological magnetization did not exist, and that mesmerism was the work of the imagination. Even today, we know little more about the nature of the hypnotic condition than did that committee of pre-revolutionary French gentlemen.

In spite of the French Royal Commission's scepticism, the phenomenon would not go away. However, the more it subsequently developed as a serious challenge to medical orthodoxy – like the roughly contemporary flowering of homeopathy – the more it was routinely denounced as 'unscientific' and 'quackery' by the (hardly more scientific) medical establishment. In the 1840s, a distinguished London doctor John Elliotson, who taught mesmerism to Dickens, attracted considerable professional odium by proselytizing the medical use of hypnosis. *The Lancet* thundered against Elliotson and 'the harlotry which he dares to call science'. Yet, apart from brandy, mesmerism was the first genuine surgical anaesthesia to be used in the Western world, and was in regular use some years before ether and chloroform were first tried in 1846 and 1847 respectively. By that time, Elliotson had chronicled seventy-six painless operations performed under mesmeric anaesthesia. Hundreds of others were done later, less publicly though rather more safely than the chemical alternatives of the age.[2] Unfortunately for hypnosis, these chemicals found immediate favour with doctors who quickly saw that such methods, however unsafe, could be far more easily contained in a scientific explanation than the always potentially embarassing legacy of Mesmer. Coincidentally, in the same month (October 1847) as the first operation under ether was performed in the United States, the distinguished British physician Sir John Forbes had called for a proper trial of anaesthetic hypnosis. Yet no sooner had the news from America been received than the *Medical Gazette* ran a headline announcing 'ANIMAL MAGNETISM SUPERCEDED'.[3]

Elliotson was a clever but flamboyant eccentric and these qualities were amply displayed in his dogged advocacy of mesmerism; probably his oddness was more hindrance than help to its future. Yet he wrote up some remarkable cases, not merely about anaesthesia but also about the wider powers of hypnosis – as it was now beginning to be called.

THE CASE OF ROSINA BARBER

She was a middle-aged spinster who consulted Elliotson in 1841 with a large lump on her breast. Elliotson's first thought was that she would need surgery and, since he found her a deeply susceptible subject, he began to prepare her for mesmeric anaesthesia. The great surgeons of the day – including James Brodie and Robert Liston – saw her, but opinion was divided as to whether the widespread tumour was operable. The cancer soon began to ulcerate, breaking through the skin, and now Elliotson determined to treat her with mesmerism alone. For long periods he put her in a state of 'happy trance', seeing her up to three times each day to re-induce her. Gradually she gained weight and strength, while the ulcerated tumour healed over and began to shrink. The improvement continued steadily, except for just one period when Elliotson was visiting the continent; during this time Miss Barber relapsed and her tumour began to grow again, until on his return Elliotson was able to resume treatment. His patient then continued to make good progress. By 1848 Elliotson reported that 'the cancerous mass is now completely dissipated, not the slightest lump is to be found nor is there the slightest tenderness of the bosom or the armpit.' Astonished that she was still alive, many of the same eminent surgeons who saw her in 1841 had already confirmed Elliotson's description.

In the light of what I have already written regarding cancer, a clue can perhaps be gleaned about Miss Barber's recovery from the phrase *'happy* trance'. But we might also speculate that in Elliotson, she found that 'significant relationship' which LeShan says is so characteristically lacking in cancer patients; or, more generally, that the abysmal loneliness of all the sick found its perfect healing answer in the constant and stalwart attentions of the hypnotherapist. Freud discovered much later that 'transference' – the process by which the patient in psycho-analysis tends to fall in love with the analyst, as Anna O. had fallen in love with Breuer – was a necessary part of the healing process. He also believed that hypnosis was itself akin to a 'loving relationship'.

What, then, can science say about hypnosis? I have said that little more is known today than in the eighteenth century, yet that little is significant for it is now established that the hypnotic trance exists. In the last ten years electro-encephalography (which measures the brain's electrical activity) has proved that the trance is distinct from both the waking and the sleeping state. The EEG of a subject being hypnotized is initially similar to that of relaxation and sleepiness but, according to the discoveries of some Soviet researchers as late as the 1970s, there is a *sudden shift* in the EEG pattern as soon as the trance state is explicitly entered; the electrical behaviour of the brain becomes different. For example, in normal consciousness the experience of smelling a flower does not register on the EEG. But if under hypnosis it is suggested that the subject smells a particularly pungent rose, there *is* a distinct EEG reaction.[4] This EEG evidence is certainly interesting, but it does not explain what a trance is or how it comes about.

The ability to hypnotize, if mysterious, is not uncommon. No special powers are needed and most people can learn to do it. One can even hypnotize oneself. When hypotizing another subject, however, the essential ingredient seems to be the practitioner's moral ascendancy. According to most authorities, this must be voluntary and yielded by the subject under conditions of absolute trust.

Classically, the hypnotist induces the subject to pay attention only to his own voice, and to shut out all other sensory inputs. As an aid to concentration there may be a spinning disc, swinging fob-watch or bright light to stare at. But the essential pathway is through the monotonous use of *words*, as F. L. Marcuse shows in an account of his technique:

> I want you to listen carefully to what I say, I want you to listen carefully to what I say, your eyes are closed, your eyes are closed, you are feeling comfortable, relaxed, thinking of nothing, nothing but what I say, your eyes are closed, comfortably closed, you are thinking of nothing, nothing but what I say . . .[5]

And so on, for another page in the paperback edition of Marcuse's book. If the induction is successful, the subject is put into a state of 'deep sound sleep' – not, of course, a conventional sleep, but a hypnotic sleep, a trance. The subject's awareness is narrowed down until it falls completely under the control of the hypnotist, who alone has access to the subject's mind and who is the only channel between the subject and the outside environment. In this state of concentrated attention, forgotten memories can be rediscovered and hidden feelings and motives can appear. Repression can also be artificially created using post-hypnotic suggestion, and *novel* motives, feelings and even memories can be implanted in the mind.

Body states can also be altered under suggestion, but not necessarily by ordering such-and-such a change. For example, you would be unlikely to induce adrenalin secretion under hypnosis by saying 'secrete adrenalin'; but if you plant the suggestion of being hunted by wolves, the 'fight-or-flight' responses will at once be evoked – including, of course, adrenalin flow. The British researcher into mind/body interaction, Stephen Black, found the same thing with blood flow. It is hard to get the blood vessels to dilate with the suggestion 'Your blood vessels are dilating' or even with 'You are hot', but it seems that if you say 'You are hot because you are standing directly in front of a huge bonfire on Guy Fawkes Night' at once the flow of blood increases and the skin reddens. This shows that the imagery of the mind and the emotional interplay involved are crucial to the effects of hypnosis. These are pure mind/body effects which cannot be explained by any version of Descartes' mechanism.

Skin conditions such as warts, acne, psoriasis and the neuro-dermatoses can often be very effectively treated by hypnosis. Here the therapy is obviously most effective if it tackles the root emotional causes, bringing about insight. Yet one of the most dramatic hypnotic cures on record was done by suggesting that the skin simply became clear. This was a case of a boy with ichthyosis reported in the *British Medical Journal* in 1952. In this condition the sweat and grease glands are fewer than normal and the skin cracks and dries up, becoming hard, scaly and often discoloured as dirt collects between the scales. Yet this boy – whose skin was grossly affected by an extreme case of the disease – turned out to be an excellent hypnotic subject and was cured under hypnosis solely by the *suggestion* of clear skin, first on his left arm only and then, progressively, over the rest of his body.[6] This is particularly hard to explain, as ichthyosis is regarded as a hereditary condition with no known emotional cause.

SURGEONS OF THE MIND

If the trance gives special access to the unconscious (by-passing the censorious ego) the reasons why hypnosis happens at all are quite unknown. Ainsley Meares, an Australian psychiatrist, has suggested it is an atavistic process – a return to a primitive state of mind. Meares thinks that before our acquisition of a brain cortex – the brain's logic-centre – the mind operated by conditioning and suggestion alone. In hypnosis, he believes, we regress to that state, progressively switching off the rationality and self-consciousness by which we normally live until our most primitive emotional levels of mind are 'exposed'.[7]

An interesting analogy gives a slightly different angle on this. Therapeutic hypnosis has been described as being like a form of 'mental surgery' where the conscious mind is put to 'sleep' by a psychic equivalent to anaesthesia – not, of course, to be confused with the *physical* anaesthesia which hypnosis can induce. The therapist is then said to 'open' the mind, folding back the defensive shield (in Freudian terms, the Ego) which guards the unconscious. Thus the hypnotist is enabled to look into the ocean depths of desire, fantasy and symbolism which contain the roots of our emotions.

Obviously, if this is true, hypnosis can be used purely to diagnose a psychological problem and bring its origin into the light. Breuer found this effective, at least temporarily, with Anna O.'s multiple symptoms; here the therapist was part investigator, part conduit for the therapeutic process – a kind of psychological homeopath, accelerating the psyche's natural healing power without introducing foreign elements into it.

However, hypnosis can be employed allopathically and it is here that the surgical analogy holds. In this case the therapist performs something very like an operation when he tries to remove or rearrange some of the contents of the unconscious, or to insert new elements into it. The purpose – as in all allopathy – is to persuade the subject's psyche back into balance.

This procedure has obvious dangers. Gordon Rattray Taylor tells of a woman who, in middle age, experienced harrowing emotional disturbances which she could neither control nor explain. In desperation she tried hypnotherapy in the hope that it might help her. As a young woman during the war she had worked at a secret military unit, but there were peculiar gaps in her memory of the period. Under hypnosis she recalled that one of her colleagues had died in distressing and controversial circumstances – but why had she so thoroughly repressed this? It took further hypnotherapy before, with great difficulty, she recovered the memory that an officer had hypnotized her and told her to forget the entire incident. As Taylor says, apart from the morality of this the lesson to draw is that 'suggestion of amnesia does not wipe out the record, it merely prevents it rising to consciousness'.[8] Therefore it seems that, like other allopathic approaches, mental surgery may be of limited use and, if misused, can be extremely harmful.

For all its mysterious 'altered states' and the arcane-sounding language of 'induction', 'suggestion', 'counter-suggestion' and so on, hypnosis is probably not an occult phenomenon but a heightened form of deference to the will of another. In medical terms, this is the process of ceasing to be an agent and becoming a patient.

Imagery

Images are products of the mind and in particular the imagination. Without the ability to make them, we could not have created our complicated human societies nor could we survive in them. Imagery both creates and sustains our myths and beliefs and is intrinsic to all creative activity. Many of these images are communal: shared mental talismans which help to stick groups of people together, like – at the most simplistic level – national flags or company logos. Individuals have personal paradigms, fruits of their own unique history, and these private images can wield an influence over their own attitudes, careers and life histories equivalent to that of the shared social images.

There are many 'talismanic' effects in medicine. Some people believe these explain the placebo effect, which becomes the result of harmony between a treatment (or perhaps just the medical team behind it) and the patient's symbolic idea of an effective agent of healing. Whether or not this holds as a *sufficient* explanation of placebo, the establishment of significant links between mental imagery and physical health would once again demonstrate the interpenetration of the body with the mind.

Perhaps the most dramatic of such effects is the *stigmata*. Much Christian meditation centres on the image of the crucified Christ, which shows five wounds: the crucifixion nail-marks in each hand and each foot and the wound of the soldier's lance in his side. Individuals who through intense meditation have achieved a high degree of identification with this image can actually reproduce these wounds in their own bodies: St Francis of Assisi carried the stigmata and so, in our own time, did the Italian Capuchin monk Padre Pio who died in 1968. The stigmata are believed by Catholics – the branch of Christianity which is most absorbed in the imagery of the crucifixion – to be marks of the highest holiness and faith and, as such, are not subjected to the indignity of scientific tests. At least one case, however, has been put through a rigorous and sceptical medical examination.

THE CASE OF LOUISE LATEAU

She was an eighteen-year-old Belgian girl who, in April 1868, had visions of the Virgin which lasted continuously for six days. Three days later, on a Friday, blood was found to be oozing from her side; the next day the flow stopped and her skin apparently cleared. On the following Friday her side bled again, and this time her feet also. A week later, the palms of her hands were affected. This went on for several months until, in due course, Lateau's forehead, too – where Christ wore the crown of thorns – began to bleed. Later still, a further area of bleeding appeared on the right shoulder, corresponding to where the cross rested during the walk to Calvary. Throughout these haemorrhages, which lasted several hours, Lateau was described as being in a state of ecstatic trance. The blood would not clot until the 'attack' was over.

Lateau continued to experience the stigmata for several years. In 1874 the Royal Academy of Belgium was sufficiently disturbed by the publicity surrounding her case to mount an investigation – in the hope of proving her a fraud, for they assumed she was secretly scratching or pricking herself and then somehow keeping the wounds open. But try as they might the Academicians could unmask no deception. When the dried scabs were removed from her palms and the skin examined under a magnifying glass, it was found to be neither punctured nor marked. Lateau was made to wear an apparatus which completely enclosed her hand and effectively prevented her from damaging it externally; nevertheless, the haemorrhage returned.

If imagery can stimulate this kind of bodily change, it is hardly surprising that it has traditionally been recognized as a powerful force in healing. It is at the basis of much of the primitive medicine which was and is still practised by those individuals recognized by their tribe as expert. These shamans are usually deliberate manipulators of imagery. For example, Navaho Indian shamans invariably used sand-painting as a central focus of their healing rituals. In many tribes, such as the Crow Indians, visualization techniques were employed to make diagnoses and seek guidance in the spirit world about treatment and prevention.[9] The integration of subjective with objective in the rituals and prayers of the shamans is what distinguishes these systems of medicine as holistic.

Many modern techniques of psychological medicine employ equivalent notions. In psychodrama, patients act out roles relevant to their condition; art therapy has well-established credentials; Jungian psychological analysis examines dreams in search of diagnostic and therapeutic insight. But these are largely restricted to conditions of the mind. Much more recently, old shamanistic practices have been tried in the hope of curing serious physical illness.

Working in Texas with cancer patients, radiologist Carl

Simonton and psychotherapist Stephanie Matthews-Simonton are pioneers of one such technique. The Simontons take seriously the idea of an emotional and a stress component in the disease process (see Chapter 6). The approach is to combine a therapeutic physical exercise – or rather, relaxation – with a mental one. The mental exercise consists of the patients using their own symbolic imagery to picture the cancer and the body's healing processes which oppose the cancer's growth and spread. This is not random 'daydreaming' but guided imagery, which means they are encouraged to generate their own images within particular frameworks: let us say by first imagining the tumour, then symbolically picturing the immune system, before watching how they interact together and so on. Even computer games have been brought in to enhance the capacity to boost up the immune system with the imagination. At the M. D. Anderson Hospital in Houston, along with their conventional chemotherapy child cancer patients play a video game called 'Killer T Cells'.

This imagery, though guided, can be highly personal – the more so the better. Brian Inglis quotes one of the Simontons' patients as saying: 'The cancer would be a snake, a wolverine or some vicious animal; the cure, white husky dogs by the millions.' When in the patient's imagination the snake shrank from the dogs and almost disappeared, 'the white army of dogs would lick up the residue and clean my abdominal cavity until it was spotless'.[10]

Jeanne Achterberg has carried out a study to see if the *quality* of the sufferer's imagery about cancer was predictive of that patient's outcome. Her research involved giving a psychological test specifically designed to record the patients' imagery and her results show that quality – the *nature* of the imagery freely generated – can be used to predict the outcome of the disease.

Archetypal figures from myth with strong protective associations such as Robin Hood, knights errant, Viking explorers etc. were strongly associated with a good outcome. Animals 'with a strong killer instinct' were popular because patients thought they *ought* to be effective, though they were only sometimes associated with a positive outcome. Those who forced such images often abandoned them because 'they got disgusted with the gore'. Imagery that was associated with a poor outcome involved:

. . . vague, weak, amorphous symbols for the immune system such as snowflakes or clouds. More often than not those with a poor prognosis couldn't draw or describe anything at all related to the immune system, but had vivid images of their cancer. A truly poor outcome was forecast when the cancer cells were seen as immutable, grasping, or ineradicable, when symbolized as lumps of coal, crabs, ants, or submarines; a better outcome was likely when they were described as weak animals or even as the actual cells as one might view them under a microscope. Interestingly enough the insect images are a grim omen of disease in the shamanistic system as well.[11]

The fact that these images correlate with how well the patient turns out does not mean that they *cause* the outcome. Achterberg does not seem to think that there is an automatic trigger in the imagination which anyone can release in order to kill cancer cells and shrink tumours. The images in themselves are more like symptoms than forms of active medication; they speak eloquently of the meaning of a disease, but they do not necessarily change it.

In actual fact, the Simontons claim better results than is normally expected from conventional treatment alone; the average survival period for their patients is said to be three times the national average for American cancer sufferers. This may indeed be because some of these patients enhance their immunity by finding effective symbolic talismans. Others have no doubt done well for different reasons; perhaps they respond to the care and attentiveness extended by the medical team, to the programme's recognition of their individuality and to the feeling of being involved in something exciting and special – all intangible elements of the kind which help to make healing an intuitive *transpersonal* affair. But if some patients *can* shrink tumours with imagery, what is it that sets them apart from others who cannot?

Meditation

I believe that the answer can be found in the fact that guided imagery is really a meditative exercise. We have already seen that for those who are capable of reaching deep trance states, meditation can achieve extraordinary changes in the body.

Yogis have been buried underground for many hours at a time – not in a box, but simply covered with a sack or plank and then with four feet of earth. They survive because they are able to reduce their physical functions, especially the need for oxygen, almost to nothing – a deliberately entered state of extreme hibernation.

Meditation also seems to be at the root of the stigmata. Louise Lateau's bleeding was always accompanied by deep trance states in which her skin became desensitized and her eyes dull and almost insensitive to light. Her body temperature and rate of breathing dropped and her pulse was lowered from 120 to 100. On coming out of her trance, she would find she had temporarily lost her own body-image, and would have to look to see where her limbs were.

Sudden and medically inexplicable cures such as have been documented at the shrine of Lourdes in southern France may derive from similar factors to those which cause stigmata – in other words, making use of imagery 'guided' by the symbolism of the sick person's Catholic faith. However this may be, it should be remembered that such cures are extremely rare. Lourdes is visited annually by hundreds of thousands of sick pilgrims of whom only a tiny proportion experience anything like a miracle – a cure which can be explained by faith alone or, in the church's terms, by divine intervention. Yet these rare examples are worth pausing over.

To receive official recognition from the church, Lourdes cures must have a number of factors in common. First, they must all refer to diagnosed forms of organic pathology; second, there must have been a sudden unexpected improvement in the condition during or shortly after visiting the shrine; third, this improvement must have been maintained until the point of substantial cure, with no relapse for three or four years; and fourth, this cure must have no acceptable medical explanation.

So Lourdes cures – if they are to be authenticated by the church – must by definition be beyond the ken of ordinary medical science. The investigations involved are carried out over a number of years by an International Medical Commission and if there is even the faintest shadow of a 'normal' – i.e. a physical or even an acceptable psychosomatic – explanation, the notion of a miracle is rejected. If adequate documentation is not available, or if the cured person's own doctor refuses to co-operate in the demanding investigations, the claims are likewise rejected. Each year an average of forty possible miracles are considered by the Lourdes Medical Bureau, the clearing house for miraculous claims, yet in the last forty years fewer than thirty miracles have been officially recognized. One of those which was recognized was that of Vittorio Micheli.

THE CASE OF VITTORIO MICHELI[12]

In April 1962 Micheli, a twenty-two-year-old conscript in the Italian Army, was admitted to hospital with pain in the lower left hip, the bone known as the left ischium. This was diagnosed as osteo-sarcoma, a malignant cancer of the bone. His condition was regarded from the outset as incurable, so that during the whole of his illness Micheli received only palliative treatment.

Within a year he was in almost continuous pain. A whole section of pelvic bone, around the place where the femur of his left leg had previously socketed into it, was eaten away. The only connection between the leg-bone and the pelvis was now 'a few sheaves of marrow', while the previously hard bone had become 'a shapeless mass, of doughy consistency'. Micheli wore a cast which for a while enabled him to walk, but by 24 May 1963 when he set out on a pilgrimage to Lourdes, his leg had become completely inert and useless.

On his return from Lourdes the doctor noted a 'sudden arrest of growth of the tumour'. One month later, Micheli could walk again. By the end of November, pain had stopped and he had significantly gained weight. Finally, just one year after the pilgrimage, the patient had been discharged from hospital and was picking up the threads of his life. He was able to do this because there had been 'remarkable reconstruction of the bony tissue of the pelvis', including the formation of a new socket into which the head of the femur fitted, thus making his leg fully functional again. He could now walk without the aid of plaster-cast or even a stick. Thus Micheli was completely rehabilitated; he married, started a family and took a job which involved working eight hours a day *standing* at a machine.

Twelve years later he was still in excellent health. The verdict of the medical panel pronounced in 1976 was that neither they nor any of the many orthopaedic surgeons they spoke to had ever encountered a spontaneous regression of malignant bone tumours, but that since Micheli had at no time received treatment intended as a cure, this must with him have been the case. They were forced to conclude that 'no medical explanation of this cure can be given'.

The procedure of investigating such cases resembles a trial, with the doctors endeavouring – like a jury – to put the matter 'beyond reasonable doubt'. The rigour of the process means that, in reality, rather more cures must occur than the figures suggest. Nevertheless, to be cured by a Lourdes pilgrimage, as Micheli was, must still be a very rare event indeed.

One of the most interesting aspects of the Micheli case is that he did not realize at once that he was cured. There was no dramatic revelation or blinding insight and he returned to the hospital from Lourdes apparently in the same physical and mental state as when he had left, encased in a plaster cast made specially strong to survive the ordeal. But in spite of his seeming unconsciousness of what had happened, my guess would be that in some way Micheli is an unusually spiritual man, with an ability to reach rare peaks of transcendence through prayer or meditation. The fact that this ability may have been hidden from the world is neither here nor there, since such attributes are necessarily private. A more publicized example was Louise Lateau; and so, of course, are many swamis and yogis. However, there must be millions of otherwise quite unremarkable people who possess heightened spiritual or meditational ability, and many of the patients who do well under the Simontons' guided-imagery cancer therapy probably fall into this category.

Most of us will never approach that kind of transcendence, perhaps because we are not inclined to or else because we are incapable. Yet more mundane and shallow acts of meditation can have useful if less dramatic effects. I have met a South London GP, Dr Chandra Patel, who has made a name for herself teaching simple mantra-meditation to patients with high blood pressure, obesity and tobacco addiction. She gets excellent results. Similar good results can come from biofeedback training, where the concentration of the mind on inner physical states is aided by the use of machinery which can tell you what is happening inside you. In this way, a blood-pressure monitor or a muscle-tension indicator linked to a fluctuating tone and fed to the patient through headphones can teach the ability to adjust the blood pressure or relax the muscles at will. Although these effects are minor, usually they alter the internal environment sufficiently to effect a desirable change in blood pressure, mental stress or whatever.

Oriental medicine

Ever since Zen became associated with motor-cycles through Robert M. Pirsig's successful book, the idea of a philosophic meeting between East and West has become part of the intellectual landscape. Many people think of this in terms of a reconciliation between two polar opposites, although such an idea does not bear too much examination.

For a start, neither Western nor Eastern thought is homogenous. The Oriental mind is as much a rag-bag of influences as the Occidental, and perhaps more so. Eastern spirituality is often taken to be the Orient's most characteristic feature, yet it has long been compromised by a fascination with the ways and means of the West. Thus, for example, the connection between yen and the marketing of motor-cycles is currently of more significance to the world than Pirsig's marriage of Zen and biking. On the other hand, it is obvious that the grand ancient cultures of Buddhism, Taoism and Hinduism are each rooted in a common approach to life which is fundamentally at odds with that of modern Europe, and that they still to an overwhelming extent shape the existence of people living anywhere between Afghanistan and Kamchatka. This is possibly more apparent today than in the past, not in spite of but because of the rapid encroachment of Western scientific materialism in the East, since this has sharpened the picture's contrast. The final effect is similar to what might have happened in Europe if the pre- and the post-Cartesian philosophies had survived together on an almost equal footing – not reconciled and certainly not merged, but sometimes co-existing in a kind of pragmatic partnership.

In medicine this is especially evident in China, where traditional healing practices are used alongside Western medicine. In fact, there is in China one notable bridge between the two traditions, since acupuncture is used as an anaesthetic for surgical operations. But in some ways this is a strange development, for to put acupuncture at the service of an alien philosophy must seem to some like a kind of prostitution.

Acupuncture is not an end in itself, nor an accidentally stumbled-across means of relief like the aspirin. It is part of an ancient and comprehensive theory of health and disease. The traditional Chinese doctor takes a history in as much minute detail as the homeopath, though there the similarity ends. The former's aim is essentially to diagnose and correct imbalances in the *energy patterns* (the *chi*) of the patient's body. *Chi* is an essential concept of traditional Chinese medicine, though to Western doctors it does not even exist. The Chinese believe that it flows through the body along certain pathways, pathways which can become blocked and cause disease. It is at intersections along these pathways that the acupuncture points are found; stimulation of these points with a probing needle is believed to stimulate the release of the *chi* and to correct the imbalances which cause disease.

The concept of *chi* is really a vitalist principle, a life-force, and such vitalism is at the heart of most forms of Oriental medicine. Instead of *chi*, Tibetan practice uses the idea of humours, which it has adapted from the ancient Greeks and interprets as the 'gross' energies of the body. Most diseases spring from imbalances in these energies and, as with Galen, treatment consists in trying to correct the imbalances.

Mention of Galen might imply that the Tibetan doctor is a primitive figure, cut off from modern life behind the high Himalayas. However, this is far from the truth despite appearances to the contrary. When the Dalai Lama's personal physician demonstrated his method at the Yale Medical Centre in Connecticut, he was allotted a patient at random and taken to her bedside. First he simply contemplated her for several minutes, then he settled down to listen to her pulse. This he did for a full *half hour* before moving on to examine a urine specimen, which he whisked with two sticks and smelt three times.

He then held a case conference with the Yale medical team, who asked for his diagnosis. He spoke of winds roaring through her body, of interrupted currents and of gates bursting open to corrupt the blood and stretch the heart. The Western medics were none the wiser, some barely concealing their smiles. Could the learned doctor give a more specific diagnosis? No problem.

'Congenital heart disease,' pronounced the robed and monk-like figure. 'Intraventricular septal defect, with resultant heart failure.'[13]

Tibetan medical philosophy is a synthesis of Chinese, Indian and Graeco-Persian elements, so it is not surprising that it should incorporate more recent Western developments into its thinking. With a view to finding out more about this, I met Dr Lopsang Rapgay, a Tibetan physician whose practice is in the medically cosmopolitan city of Delhi. Dr Rapgay is not critical of Western medicine; to him it is simply another system which people will take up or abandon according to its usefulness. When I asked him if he recognized the existence of the placebo effect, he answered that indeed he did; it was something that the traditional Tibetan doctor will deliberately try to evoke by using imagery and attention, while at the same time employing a more orthodox therapy. He told me:

> Cancer, certainly terminal cancer, cannot be treated by purely mechanical means. So in a traditional clinic the doctor will ask the client to visualize him (the doctor, I mean) as a deity, as the Buddha of medicine. And while he performs the treatment, which is basically heat therapy on the tumour, he evokes certain emotions in the client whereby he sees the doctor as an external force and that the treatment is being carried out through that medium.

The use of that particular imagery is of course specific to those who can make *use* of the Buddha of medicine. The response, if it comes, is personal and psychological; it cannot be imposed from outside.

I do not use the term 'complementary' medicine, because in many ways these therapies are too starkly contrasted with the thinking behind orthodox Western medicine to be able to complement it. However, the essential points of contrast with orthodoxy are also those which give the alternatives discussed in this chapter a family resemblance to each other. I would summarize these essences as follows:

1. Every illness is treated as a unique event.
2. The healer forms a diagnosis by means of close *attentiveness* to the patient as an individual.

3. Therapy aims to draw out the patient's latent powers of self-healing.
4. There is assumed to be no separation between organic, psychological and spiritual factors in the origin of the disease, or in its treatment.

Any of the alternative medical systems I have discussed can be used as a vehicle for mystical or spiritual beliefs, but to do so is usually to exaggerate that side of their nature. Certainly they pay attention to the spiritual side of life, but this is merely common sense since that aspect exists and is important. Yet these are *practical* strategies for coping with illnesses, and it is this essential simplicity and practicality which has ensured their survival. What is the source of their power? I believe it is the same as the power which also appears – in attenuated form – in Western medicine under the name placebo. Dr Rapgay himself believes this of the medicine he practices, but he does not therefore feel ashamed of his profession, as if he were committing some kind of systematic fraud. For him, to evoke placebo *is the whole point of his work*:

> The basic factor which sustains human beings is the ability to operate with a sense of trust, and to harness that trust. In a basically hostile environment, you need to be able to believe that there is some energy in the body to help you. You need the ability to activate and motivate yourself to see yourself through.

There could hardly be a better restatement of the conditions, sketched in the last chapter, for the effective operation of placebo effect.

Chapter 11

The whole story

'. . . But first, the notion that man has a body
distinct from his soul is to be expunged'
William Blake

A familiar but, for all that, a powerful criticism of the scientific
outlook is that it has carved a split in our perception of the
world, a deep and damaging split between the objectivity of
logic and the subjectivity of our experience. I have already
pointed out a number of ways in which this affects our attitudes
to medicine: it is, for example, clearly shown in the feelings and
opinions which Jocelyn Cornwell discovered in Bethnal Green.

That poets and artists were among the first to articulate this
criticism of objectivity is not surprising. Our sense of ourselves
as something more than machines comes largely from sources
deep within us, which float up from the depths of the unconscious ocean. And as Freud said, 'It was not I but the poets
who discovered the unconscious.' The poet and mystic William
Blake's 'Marriage of Heaven and Hell' [1] is as powerful a mani-
festo as you could have for the belief that the impulse of objectivity is inherently tyrannical. Blake, like Freud, was a great
believer in oppositions. 'Without Contraries,' he said, 'there is
no progression.' In keeping with this view, he was himself a
polemicist of tireless – and to some of his contemporaries, tire-
some – gifts.

One of the contraries Blake perceived was that existing
between the creative forces, the sources of energy in the
Universe and the 'Devouring' forces which negate energy. Blake
says: 'To the Devourer it seems as if the producer (of energy)
was in his chains; but it is not so, he only takes portions of

existence and fancies it the whole.' For Blake the chains were those of Newtonian reason, which believed itself all-comprehending and capable of a complete domination of nature. Other Romantic writers followed Blake in asserting the primacy of nature over 'the Ratio'.

When Wilhelm Reich, an unashamed romantic psychologist, wrote that 'the more one is caught up in the toils of dependency, the louder one claims to be an "objective scientist" ' [2] he was articulating the same insight but reversed: illusions of objectivity concealing the addictive delusions of grandeur.

The Newtonian and Cartesian views of reality still dominate biology and medicine. The effect of this on doctors and scientists is itself potentially injurious, since it involves an unnatural split between themselves as scientists and as people. The fact that hundreds of physicists could coldly and methodically work day after day, year after year on the calculations required to construct the first nuclear bomb – when they were the only people with a clear idea of what it would do – is a tribute to the human psyche's capacity to be split and yet still function, like a worm cut in half.

But it can be extremely disconcerting if, suddenly, the precarious set of illusions needed to sustain this situation is punctured. A powerful instance occurs in a medical context in Alexander Solzhenitsyn's *Cancer Ward*. Ludmila Dontsova, one of the hospital's senior cancer specialists, is an excellent doctor, pursuing her duty of objectivity with strict dedication:

> Etiology, pathogenesis, symptoms, diagnosis, the course of the disease, treatment, prevention, prognosis – all these were real enough. The doctor might have sympathy with the patients' resistance, doubts and fears; these were understandable human weaknesses, but they didn't count for anything when it came to deciding which method should be used. There was no place left for such feelings in the squares of logic.

But Dontsova must now face the diagnosis of her own cancer:

> Until now all human bodies had been built identically as described in the standard anatomical atlas. The physiology of the vital processes and the physiology of sensations were uniform as well. Everything that was normal or deviated from the normal was explained in logical terms by authoritative manuals.

Then suddenly, within a few days, her own body had fallen out of this great orderly system. It had struck the hard earth and was now like a helpless sack crammed with organs – organs which might at any moment be siezed with pain and cry out.

Within a few days everything had been turned inside out. Her body was, as before, composed of parts she knew well, but the whole was unknown and frightening.[3]

In literature, occasions when the biter is bit are usually kept for comic or satirical effect. When such reversals are reported by Fleet Street, on the other hand, they are 'ironic', except in cases of death or fatal illness when they are 'tragic'. Solzhenitsyn aims for a more genuine measure of tragedy than popular journalism comprehends, but there is of course an element of political and social satire here, too. Dontsova, an efficient and dedicated functionary who is used to dealing with patients as aggregates of their organic parts, has forgotten (or never learned) how to comprehend even herself as a whole person. If nations, too, are governed by reductionist philosophies, can we believe their rulers capable of real humanity? Dontsova is no tyrant, but she is an unwitting agent of the same 'devouring' negation which Blake had attacked.

However, while medicine today has a well-developed negative side, one should put these in perspective: the worst excesses of clinical tyranny are not committed in these high-tech times. Witness Blake's own quite horrific burlesque description of a surgeon at work in a London charity hospital, written in about 1787:

He'll plunge his knife up to the hilt in a single drive, and thrust his fist in, and all in the space of a quarter of an hour. He does not mind their crying though they cry ever so. He'll swear at them and keep them down with his fist & tell them that he'll scrape their bones if they don't lay still and be quiet. What the devil should the people in the hospital that have it done for nothing make such a piece of work for?[4]

The rift between the scientific and the personal afflicted official medicine even before the eighteenth century. Indeed, King James's translator of the *Book of Ecclesiasticus* must have been thinking of a doctor similar to Blake's when he wrote: 'He that sinneth before his Maker, let him fall into the hand of the

Physician.' Yet in many ways, the Biblical view of illness has advantages. I must quickly say that I am not advocating a return to the equation of disease with sin, but would simply point out that the idea does at least envisage a humanity in which moral and physical life interpenetrate one another. With its moral superstructure and substructure of emotions, the mind and the spirit inform and are informed by our physical life. It is not clear to me how they can do so if posted by Gilbert Ryle into an entirely different logical pigeonhole from the physical. Mind works through meaning and meaning must be communicated. The idea of communication between the moral, the mental and the physical makes sense only within a holistic framework, and not at all within a mechanistic one.

The meaning of illness

Disease is not an episode of foreign domination, as I hope has become clear by now. It is a medium of meaning and, as such, it can be no more alien to us than speech, and obviously less so than clothes or architecture. What it has in common with all these is its highly personal and at the same time deeply social significance: that there are 'maladies which speak'. Such an idea is resisted by mechanical medicine to the best of its ability and, though it can never completely exclude the personal element, its desire to do so is much enhanced by its mastery of drugs and high technology. The trouble is that abolishing symptoms with drugs is like responding to a chalked distress message with a blackboard duster.

From the start, I have emphasized this meaningfulness of illness. Should I not say instead that all *symptoms* have meaning? In conventional medical philosophy one of the first duties of the physician is to distinguish symptoms and signs from the disease itself. This is diagnosis. It is all a matter of reading the meaning of symptoms, and it is always spoken of as almost an intuitive process or even an art, although interpretative rather than creative – piano-playing rather than composing. Before they could do much therapeutic good, this function was taken very seriously by doctors, although they had other and even more important duties. As the American physician Lewis Thomas has pointed out in a recent autobiography, the medical

221

training he received in the 1920s emphasized that 'what the ill patient and his family wanted most was to know the name of the illness, and then, if possible, what had caused it and finally, most important of all, how it was likely to turn out'.[5]

Telling the name of a disease is always a start, because it elucidates the meaning of symptoms – that bulging eyes indicate a thyroid condition and yellow skin (jaundice) a liver disease. In this perspective, the meaning carried by symptoms is always the existence of underlying disease. (I am here using the word 'symptom' in its lay sense of 'a manifestation of disease' rather than in its rather more restricted medical sense of 'that which the patient reports'.) But the states underlying the symptoms, the 'pathological states' are themselves devoid of meaning: they are taken simply to exist.

Yet there is an inherent problem in these distinctions. In his poem 'Among School Children', W. B. Yeats could not tell the dancer from the dance: can we seriously consider distancing symptom from disease? To me, a symptomless disease is like a puddle with no water – at best a Zen joke. The manifestations of disease *are* the disease; their meaning is the disease's meaning.

However, talking at the level of symptoms (the signs; what-you-can-see) does not exhaust the meaning of illness. To deal with meaning in medicine, as Oliver Sacks says,[6] is to take on a two-fold responsibility. First of all there is identification, which employs physiology and biochemistry in a mechanical way to arrive at a rational diagnosis. But symptoms and diseases are not simply tagged with meaning as if they were plants in a garden centre. Sacks reminds us that there is a second responsibility towards meaning in disease, that of *understanding* – an activity of an entirely different order. Understanding demands reference to the whole picture, to the subjective as well as the objective, to intangibles as well as hard facts. It entails involvement in the patient's person – nature, tastes, history, personality, prejudices, fears – all the things which make him or her an individual and *different*. Mechanical medicine, on the other hand, deals by preference with interchangeable components.

The orthodox view also sees disease not as personal but as *alien* – tumours as Martian invaders and so on – a view from which the logical (if extreme) extension is 'that one must *attack* disease with all the weapons one has, and that one can launch the attack with total impunity, without thought of the person who is ill'.[7]

Such objectification of the disease and of the patient can undoubtedly be justified in purely pragmatic terms at the very extremes of emergency and life saving, when time forbids niceties. But the more general application of objectivity is also regarded as a way to guarantee fairness and avoid error. Yet in practice it does not always work out like that. One could point to individual cases such as that of Mrs Ross (p. 21) or to the outright abuse of political psychiatry as seen in the Soviet Union and elsewhere. Fairness, too, is subjectively assessed on both sides of the patient/doctor divide.

Most doctors, however scientifically oriented, concede that subjectivity is a factor in their calculations. But, like the placebo effect, it is often treated as a nuisance to be endured. Medicine, runs the argument, is a 'soft' science, in which a clear hard picture of physical reality is difficult or impossible to obtain on account of interference from personal factors. 'Hard' sciences, by contrast, have no such disadvantage; they are free to pursue objectivity regardless. On this view objectivity in medicine is still an ideal, but an unattainable one. The issue then becomes a matter of how to get near it. You want to form a picture of reality close to that of 'hard' science and as humanely as possible. The trouble is that the question, 'How near can you get?' may find itself reformulated as, 'How far can you go . . . and get away with it?'

But the use of objectivity as an ideal to aim at carries a more fundamental problem. The 'hard' sciences, which provide the model of the ideal, are themselves now beginning to abandon it and go soft – if by 'soft', we mean penetrated by subjectivity. As the psychologist Harold J. Morovitz has put it, biology and physics are two trains on the same line but travelling in opposite directions:

What has happened is that biologists who once postulated a privileged role for the human mind in nature's hierarchy, have been moving towards the hard-core materialism that characterizes nineteenth-century physics. At the same time physicists, faced with compelling experimental evidence, have been moving away from the strictly mechanical models of the universe to a view that sees mind as playing an integral role in all physical events'.[8]

The consequence of the 'compelling experimental evidence' is that the whole notion of objectivity in science is coming slowly to pieces. We can see this most obviously in the apparently absurd world of quantum physics.

In this century, modern physics has had to come to terms with a few concepts which previously were anathema to those brought up with Newtonian thought – which is the kind of thought now at the root of everyday common sense. As most people know, the first of these revolutionary concepts was relativity. It was followed by the even more disturbing principle of *uncertainty*, which principle is at the heart of quantum physics.

Uncertainty arises from difficulties in discussing the nature of matter at very low levels of magnitude – initially the electrons which orbit the nucleus of an atom, and then the protons and neutrons forming the nucleus itself. Upon investigation, these particles (and also the particle which is one aspect of light and which Einstein called the *quantum*) turn out to have a dual aspect – to be simultaneously capable of behaving like waves or like *particles*, depending on what the scientist is looking for.

This is partly an extension of Einstein's famous equation $e=mc^2$, which established that matter and energy were aspects of each other. What was new was the notion that the status of, say, an electron – whether wave-like or particle-like – *depends on the observer and on the kind of question the observer is asking*. Indeed until the question *is* asked, the electron is regarded by quantum science as being in a hybrid (or uncertain) state of existence – just like the physicist Schrodinger's famous cat. According to quantum physics, if this unfortunate animal is shut in a box and, by the random action of a quantum effect, given a fifty-fifty chance of being gassed or not gassed, it immediately becomes suspended in an in-between state – *neither* alive *nor* dead – until an observer opens the box.

This is not fancy metaphysics or a piece of paradoxical word-play. It can be demonstrated by a real experiment that the quantum is a dual personality whose behaviour – whether as a wave or a particle – depends on the act of observation alone. Even Einstein himself could not accept all the implications of uncertainty, saying that God does not play dice. But as we have noted, the revolutionary concept is not merely that subatomic nature consists of random events. It appears to require a mind to make it come into being. Said Nils Bohr, the great physicist and friend of Einstein, 'Anyone who is not shocked by quantum theory does not understand it.' Einstein's resolute opposition to uncertainty is slightly surprising, in that he himself was one of the first to introduce the observer into physics when he asked the question, 'What does reality look like to someone travelling at the speed of light?' – the question which resulted in his relativity theory. However, in relativity the role of the observer is quite passive. This new subjectivity brings the observer, and even his intention, into the picture as *active* agencies. As the physicist and Nobel prize-winner Eugene Wigner has written, 'It was not possible to formulate the laws of quantum physics without reference to the consciousness.'

It seems inevitable that eventually, and in spite of the modern biologist's (and doctor's) attachment to mechanical materialism, we will find this new physics beginning to inform a new biology. There are already signs of this: many of the quantum physicists themselves, including Schrodinger and Heisenberg, have written about the philosophical implications of quantum theory. Max Born, another important figure in the history of the quantum, said, 'I am now convinced that theoretical physics is actual philosophy' – a case of the wheel coming round to science's first origin in 'natural philosophy'. If philosophy leads, science may follow. Rupert Sheldrake's book *A New Science of Life* – candidate for burning though it may be – is another straw in the wind.

Paradigms

Observing that all systems of thought are supported by pre-existing moral assumptions, Thomas Kuhn has argued in his book *The Structure of Scientific Revolutions* that there is an intellectual relativity in the scientific world, which is thereby dependent on the assumptions or paradigms held within the scientific community. Any change in the paradigms leads ultimately to a scientific revolution. Put simply, this means that scientific findings are never absolute, that the 'truth' scientists strive for is a subjectively formulated goal which is superseded not necessarily by better measuring instruments, but by changes in the climate of thought. 'Objectivity' is therefore an illusion.

The paradigms on which mechanistic science was erected in

the seventeenth century can be illustrated by the views of Francis Bacon (1561–1626), the philosopher who laid down the ground rules for the experimental method in science. Bacon's assumptions were often violent and patriarchal. Nature was female and mysteriously threatening (a common view of the female, as I have already described in Chapter 4), so Bacon urges the need to 'torture nature's secrets from her', to 'hound' her and make her man's 'slave'. It was a perpetual struggle for, as Bacon says elsewhere, 'Nature is often hidden, sometimes overcome, seldom extinguished.' This paradigm of the manly scientific spirit struggling to dominate mother nature has remained with 'objective' science ever since, and left a strong imprint on medicine.

These paradigms, determining our notions of true and effective medicine, can be seen, in Jonathan Miller's phrase, as 'principles of symbolic potency'. The idea that effective medicine hinges on the power of its symbolism is perhaps another way to describe the importance of placebo effect. The paradigms of medicine must coincide with the symbols and ideas which we hold to be powerful in everyday life, or our confidence in it will fail. Thus, as Miller speculates, if patients in westernized societies are beginning to turn away from scientific medicine, 'it is not necessarily because they are dissatisfied with its results, but because they no longer accept the rationale on which it is based'.[9]

But it is much too early to talk about a widespread shift in paradigms. However uneasy the developed world may begin to feel about Bacon's project of suppressing and punishing nature, we are still largely dominated by it. After all, as citizens we continue to accept the large-scale release of industrial pollution. The steady destruction of forests and the extinction of wildlife proceeds with hardly a murmur of protest from most of us, as does the accumulation of nuclear, chemical and biological weaponry – although we know this to be so destructive that life on earth can hardly expect to survive an all-out third world war.

In the same way the patriarchal urge to bring nature to book, to confine and re-educate and establish power over her, is still very strong in medicine. We may no longer countenance female circumcision or frontal lobotomy as legitimate medical techniques, but spare-part surgery, test-tube reproduction, genetic

226

engineering and certain forms of aggressive chemotherapy would not have been developed and come into use without the sanction of the Baconian spirit. It seems possible that these latter procedures may one day seem as barbaric as the former. But for the moment we tend to accept that the grand object of public health policy is to push such 'progressive research' ever onwards.

In fact, as patients, we find ourselves in a curious half-way position. Although we have begun, to some extent, to reach out towards new symbolic potencies in medicine, we are a long way from grasping them with any conviction and, in spite of our unease about scientific medicine, we continue to register with mechanistic doctors, take out health insurance, and blindly sign consent forms. The same, of course, goes for our attitude to industry and the military. We fear pollution and the arms race, and yet we are consumers and citizens of nation states, and as such appear stranded like whales on a beach, at considerable political and existential distance from the endorsement of radical change.

Where can we go to break out? The most extreme ecological position I can imagine would abhor intervention of any kind in nature. This will hardly do since the result is a kind of bovine anarchism, by which no tree would ever be cut, nor house built, nor loaf of bread baked nor wound dressed. But when Gerard Manley Hopkins lamented the loss of a favourite group of trees in the poem 'Binsey Poplars', he put his finger on the central issue:

> O if we but knew what we do
> When we delve and hew –
> Hack and rack the growing green!

The plea here is not that no tree should ever be felled, but that none should be felled mindlessly, without *knowing what we do*. Knowing what we do is not the arrogant manipulations of the Baconian experimenter, however skilful. Knowing what we do is the all-round understanding which the world so urgently needs now – in economics, farming, industry, military planning. It is needed no less in education and medicine, the domestic specialisms, for it signals an understanding of the interpenetration of mind and body, of how both imagination and reason participate in the processes of life, growth, illness and death.

Finale

In this chapter I have approvingly quoted William Blake, Hopkins, Reich and Solzenitsyn, all in their own ways mystics and romantics. But our image of romanticism is of something impossibly remote and particularly impractical. This is a mistaken image but a tenacious one and, since I am arguing that something like a spirit of neoromanticism will be a necessary paradigm for any holistic medicine, the question arises what *practical* results do I expect to follow?

First of all, we are not about to witness any sudden upsurge in the use or effectiveness of self-medicine. We have always dosed ourselves for minor ailments and will continue to do so; but for many of our ills, and especially for major diseases we shall continue to need to become patients.

However, we shall also need something of a more personal (or *transpersonal*) nature than is on offer at the moment. Eventually we shall want to be more actively engaged in what happens to our bodies, especially when we undertake any therapy. This may perhaps involve something like a *partnership* with doctors and nurses. But it will require a tremendous shift in attitude amongst both patients and the medical professions and, although this is already happening here and there, such a change will only come when people are ready. They will not become so overnight, as can be clearly seen from Jocelyn Cornwell's work in Bethnal Green.

In any event, it would be useful if doctors took a lead. The doctor's *time* is the first requirement, and the re-establishment of trust – which is always supposed to have been the hallmark of the family doctor. Not all the blame for the distrust of medicine in advanced countries is due to the attitudes of doctors and health professionals. The switch to consumerism in medicine is not markedly different from the switch to consumerism in every other field of activity, including religion. However, medicine has undoubtedly either encouraged or facilitated the change. The arrival of the consumer-model in medicine has been an opportunity to boost the profession's high-technology aspirations and has also complemented the tendency of medicine to divide into specialized sub-sections. However, consumerism is entirely inappropriate for medicine and there are signs (such as the recent formation of the British Holistic Medical Association) that in some quarters the penny has dropped.

Secondly, new health services should be smaller in scale than we have seen up to now. There has already been criticism of mega-hospitals, though this has been made as much on economic as on medical grounds. In America rocketing medical costs have already caused medicine to turn a degree or two towards out-patient services, but again largely as a result of pressure from health paymasters (insurance companies and industrial corporations). This has been accepted by medicine because of technological advances: there is a rhyme going round to the effect that, 'Better local anaesthesia/Makes out-patient surgery easier'. There will perhaps need to be a more appropriate rationale than that if more local and effective medical services are to become widespread.

In Britain, where patient opinion is not effectively martialled into pressure groups, it nevertheless seems that long-standing dissatisfaction with creeping centralization is having an effect. These days there is some emphasis on General Practice in medical training (there never used to be), and the GP system is itself a remnant of the old 'family doctor' tradition – much restricted and abused, but still something on which a genuinely transpersonal health care might conceivably be based.

My third and last point follows on from this. Medicine will need to show unequivocally that it appreciates the personal nature of health and health care, and can make a stand on that principle. In many ways it is hard to see how this will come about. In mass society power is increasingly expressed in the currency of objective information, much of it scientific and technological. This is a power which can really hurt people, and with a potential to cause suffering and sickness on a grand scale. Whether it is to be brought into perspective and under human control is a political choice, but unless that happens I find it hard to see how the inner-city malaise – the condition of frustrated subjectivity expressed through crime and violence, or escaped from by means of drugs, alcohol and solvents – will not spread inexorably.

Medicine does not cure our social ills, though it spends a

great deal of time and money demonstrating this obvious fact. Yet the medical professions cannot avoid some responsibility. The 'managed maintenance of life on high levels of sub-lethal illness', the misguided use of large-scale drug therapy, the concentration on the parts rather than the whole, the turning-away from subjectivity: these will all, I think, one day be seen as denials of the meaning of illness, comparable even to those well-meaning measures of censorship which deny freedom of expression in the interests of a spurious moral security. What both denials do is empty the self of its contents. For my part I hope – with the romantics – that love can somehow come through. If on the inside of humanity there is nothing but solipsistic absurdity, there is likely to be little on the outside but automatism.

W. H. Auden put it better: 'The first anthropological axiom of the Evil One is not *All men are evil*, but *All men are the same*; and his second? *Men do not act; they only behave*.'

Postscript: AIDS – a suitable case for science?

AIDS is now regarded as the greatest peacetime medical emergency since the Spanish Flu epidemics which followed the First World War. It is much too early to say anything useful or detailed about the moral or mental component in AIDS and for this reason it has not been discussed in the main body of this book. Nevertheless, in the few years since it first appeared, this terrible disease has already brought medicine to a new watershed, and it cannot go entirely unnoticed.

AIDS is actually an acute embarrassment to scientific medicine. For one thing, it has come out of the blue, a new affliction, utterly without medical precedent and medical warning. For another, medicine has lost control of the terms under which AIDS is discussed. Debate on AIDS has not been contained within the journals and conferences of medical science, nor confined to its own obfuscatory jargon. It has invaded political, industrial and family life; it is discussed in the popular press, speculated about in bars and laundromats, and analysed from the pulpit. It has even, incredibly, moved senior police officers to pronounce on its origins. AIDS has burst the straitjacket of medical discourse, and it will be a hard struggle to wrestle it back in.

In fact, the outbreak of AIDS has shown just how flimsily we give our allegiance to the scientific account of disease. Spurred by growing concern, and receiving little reassurance from doctors and official health agencies, people have cast their nets widely for the meaning of this horror. Some, as is well known, have reverted to medieval notions of sin and divine retribution, and, although this is still no doubt the response of a small minority, most people have been forced to go some way beyond the normal field of scientific explanation in their search for the meaning of AIDS. As the disease touches more and more individuals – and I am speaking here about members of developed, predominantly white nations – the rift between personal and scientific meanings becomes wider.

The incompleteness of the information available from medical research merely discourages people from putting faith in scientific logic. First, we know that AIDS appeared initially amongst blacks, homosexuals and drug addicts, groups that are already the focus for the irrational fears and prejudices of the 'normal' majority. Since we have no idea why it first appeared in this way, the road is open for a surge of racist and homophobic rhetoric, fuelled by AIDS panic. Scientists and humanists rightly condemn this, but they have little to offer in its place.

Next, AIDS has proved to be largely a sexually transmitted disease, so that it touches our subjective lives in an even more intimate way than other sickness, and comes to resemble syphilis as it afflicted the human race between the sixteenth and nineteenth centuries. This sexual, subjective element merely fuels the insecurity which the disease provokes, an insecurity against which, as yet, science is once again largely helpless. On the other hand, it is the kind of insecurity which authoritarian politicians like to exploit.

But the main reason why AIDS is especially hard to reckon with – much harder than syphilis, cancer, heart disease or any disabling condition – is in the nature of its effect on the body-mind. AIDS means the gradual destruction of the immune system, which as we saw in Chapter 5 is the most important homeostatic principle of the body-mind, for it is no less than the cornerstone of our physical integrity. If we can no longer draw the bounds of what we are, we begin to dissolve, as if in an acid bath. Instress, the essential condition of life, is withdrawn and the individual dies under a welter of different degenerative and opportunistic diseases. This is what AIDS does, and unless checked it seems likely to do it on a very large scale indeed.

As a potent mixture of prejudiced misinformation, sexual fear and existential horror, it can be seen how AIDS introduces new symbolic potencies into the medical sphere. It also exposes the old paradigms of medical research to a most unflattering light. The sight of research centres in Paris and Washington, quarrelling over which has the right to exploit the virus commercially has not been edifying. Nor has the sound of various research centres worldwide trumpeting news of miracle drugs, many of which have been useless.

However, having said all this, I believe that *eventually*, medical science will come up with both an effective treatment for AIDS and with a vaccine. I say this because, however much damage its reputation may have sustained in the meantime, this is exactly the sort of disease with which science can deal best, as it did triumphantly in conquering syphilis, pneumonia and polio. Indeed the conquest of AIDS will at a stroke reverse the decline in the reputation of mechanistic medicine, and this in turn will give a fillip to humanity's confidence that science can one day fully comprehend all the many chronic and fatal diseases discussed above.

This revival will be real, but temporary. For in terms of the subject of this book, the search for an AIDS *cure* appears, in the long perspective, rather like a noisy and attention-getting side show. The sudden appearance of the Human Immunodeficiency Virus has been more like an environmental disaster than any of the chronic pathologies which I have been describing (though because of its effect on the immune system, it does give rise to some of these pathologies). Nevertheless, alongside the questions of the scientists, as they seek to arrest the AIDS pathogen's activity and to make us immune from its effects, the holistic questions remain. What distinguishes those carriers of the virus who do not proceed to the full-blown syndrome from those who do? What determines the speed by which the syndrome appears? Of those suffering from AIDS, who – if any – will recover spontaneously, and why? And how can AIDS sufferers be best cared for? In giving rise to such questions AIDS is no different from any of the infectious diseases which have wracked humanity. Long after the present epidemic has become a distant historical memory, they are questions which will stand.

References

Introduction

1. Quoted by Medawar, 1984
2. Wingate, 1979. Article on 'Fatigue'
3. Bateson, 1979

Chapter 1

1. Ewbank, 1842 pp 257–8
2. See Bernal, 1952
3. Quoted by Veith, 1965
4. Shorter, 1986 p 233
5. Case reported in letter to *The Lancet* 1st March 1986 pp 501–2
6. 9th November 1985 p 1048
7. 11th January 1986 p 96
8. *British Medical Journal* 1978 2 1061–2
9. Rose and Marmot, 1981
10. Quoted by Gardner, 1965 p 37
11. Abbott *et al*, 1985
12. Quoted by Wood, 1986
13. Inglis, 1981 p 8
14. *The Lancet* 10th May 1986 pp 1077–8
15. Lewis, 1961

Chapter 2

1. Miller, 1978 pp 32–3.
2. Descartes, 1968 p 165
3. This case and the next are quoted by Melzack and Wall, 1982 (Chapter 4)
4. Walters, 1961
5. Melzack and Wall, 1982 p 30
6. Mitchell, 1984 p 171
7. Freud, 1938 p 129
8. The incident occurs in chapter 1 of Powell, 1951

9. This is brilliantly discussed in Douglas, 1970
10. Speaking during a BBC television programme on Lawrence, 1986
11. Readers who think I have dodged the issue of masochism and feminism should read Maria Marcus's unique and soul-baring book. Marcus, 1981
12. 'Y', 1975

Chapter 3

1. Leviticus 13
2. Walker, 1978 p 157
3. Comments from patients writing to *Beyond The Ointment*, the journal of the Psoriasis Association
4. Champion, 1986
5. *British Medical Journal* 1985 **291**, 1523
6. Schilder, 1964 p 238
7. *ibid* p 231
8. *ibid* p 238
9. Jung 1967 p 201
10. Groddeck, 1949
11. Seville and Martin, 1981
12. Many are cited by Seville, 1983
13. Seville, 1977, 1978
14. Champion, 1986
15. Seville, 1983
16. Seville, 1978
17. Erikson, 1965 p 274
18. Updike, 1985
19. Updike, 1980
20. *The Listener* 20th November 1986

Chapter 4

1. Suttie, 1963 p 20
2. Cornwell, 1984
3. *ibid* p 131
4. *ibid* p 161
5. *NACK* January 1981
6. *NACK* Autumn 1983
7. Pfeffer and Woollett, 1983 p 47
8. *ibid* p 56
9. Taylor, 1979 p 48
10. For much of this information I am indebted to Taylor, 1979 Chapter 17
11. *The Guardian*, 15th December 1986 p 12

12. Article by A. Cabau and M. de Senarclens in Insler and Lunenfeld ed., 1986
13. *New Scientist* 6th November 1986 p 53
14. Harrison, 1984 p 153–4

Chapter 5

1. Mulhalen and Wright, 1983
2. Boswell, 1930 p 9
3. McNeill, 1979 p 235
4. Halsband, 1956 p 111
5. *ibid* p 90
6. Simeons, 1960
7. Article by Plaut and Friedmann in Ader ed., 1981
8. *New Scientist* 24 April, 1986
9. Ellis, 1898 p 180
10. *The Guardian* 5th September 1986
11. Proust, 1983 p 50
12. Maurois, 1962 p 96
13. *ibid* p 78
14. Sacks, 1981. Case no. 18
15. *ibid*. Case no. 62

Chapter 6

1. Figures from Bodley Scott, 1979
2. Bodley Scott, 1979 p 13 (italics added)
3. *ibid* p 3
4. Ader ed., 1981. Chapter 2
5. LeShan, 1984 pp 76–78
6. Article by Rosch in Cooper ed., 1984
7. Article by Temoshok and Heller, *ibid*
8. S. Greer, 1979
9. LeShan, 1984 Chapter 8
10. One of the Gnostic Gospels quoted by Elaine Pagels, 1982 p 135. Elsewhere she notes that the early Christian gnostic movement resembled modern psychotherapy in that they both 'value, above all, knowledge – the self-knowledge which is insight. They agree that, lacking this, a person experiences the sense of being driven by impulses he does not understand.' (p 133) In addition, she says, 'both agree – against orthodox Christianity – that the psyche bears *within itself* the potential for liberation or destruction.'
11. Article in Ader ed., 1981

Chapter 7

1. Jacques Lacan: 'Intervention on Transference'. Essay in Bernheimer and Kahane ed., 1985
2. Plato, 1965 p 120
3. G. Greer, 1970 p 249
4. Millett 1971 p 249
5. Plato 1965 p 120
6. Entralgo, 1955, p 116
7. *ibid* pp 117–8
8. Shorter 1984 p 287
9. Jones 1964 p 174
10. Veith, 1965
11. 7th June 1986 p 1317
12. DHSS *Social Security Statistics*, 1981
13. Fisher, 1980 p 29
14. This account follows that of Fisher *loc. cit.*

Chapter 8

1. Interviewed by *The Guardian* 23rd April 1986
2. Francois Jacob, quoted by Monod, 1974 p 29
3. Hopkins, 1966 p 127
4. *Tales from Paradise* BBC Radio Four, 1986
5. Rivers, 1920
6. Tuchman 1979 p 259
7. Inglis, 1981 p 210
8. Durden-Smith and de Simone, 1983 p 180
9. Bronowski, 1973 p 395
10. McDougall quoted by Sheldrake, 1983 p 190
11. This is movingly described in Sacks, 1976
12. Eye-witness accounts of Hitler's last days in the bunker portray a man unmistakeably siezed by the end-stage of the disease. See Fest, 1977 1079–1080
13. Sacks, 1976 p 32
14. *ibid* p 39
15. McNeill, 1979 p 264
16. Parish, 1979
17. McEvedy and Beard, 1970
18. Quoted by Karlins and Andrews, 1975 p 20
19. Taylor 1979 p 134

Chapter 9

1. Miller, 1978 p 50
2. Donne *Devotions* Chapter 21

3. One such was Dr Oliver Sacks. See Sacks, 1986
4. Koestler, 1980 p 499
5. Shorter, 1986 Chapter 6
6. Lucas, 1981 p 55
7. Cobb, 1959
8. Cited by Taylor, 1979 p 85
9. Williams, 1967 p 292
10. Sacks, 1986 p 30
11. *The Lancet*, 2nd November 1985 p 1002
12. Quoted by Carter, 1979
13. *The Guardian* 6th August 1986 p 11
14. Illich, 1977 p 42
15. Sacks, 1986

Chapter 10

1. *The Lancet*, 18th October 1981 p 881
2. Waxman, 1981 p 11
3. Tuke, 1884 p 41
4. Waxman *op. cit.* pp 35–6
5. Marcuse, 1959 p 52
6. Mason, 1952
7. Waxman *op. cit.* pp 26–7
8. Taylor, 1979 p 100
9. Achterberg, 1985 pp 48–9
10. Inglis, 1981 p 95
11. Achterberg, *op. cit.* pp 191–2
12. An appendix in Marnham, 1980, reprints in full the Micheli dossier, as compiled by the Lourdes Medical Bureau.
13. The story is told by the American doctor and writer Richard Selzer, quoted by Kaptchuk and Croucher, 1986

Chapter 11

1. Blake, 1927 p 192ff
2. Reich, 1968 p 183
3. Solzenitsyn, 1970 p 519
4. From Blake's satirical prose work *An Island in the Moon* Blake, 1927 p 865
5. Thomas, 1984 p 28
6. Sacks, 1976 p 263
7. *ibid* p 265
8. Morovitz, 1982
9. Miller, 1978 p 58

Bibliography

Books are dated according to the year of the editions consulted

Abbot J., Sutherland C., and Watt D., 'Physiological and Cognitive Responses of Type A and Type B Individuals During Academic Stress'. Paper presented to the Annual Meeting of the British Psychological Society, December 1985

Achterberg, Jeanne, *Imagery in Healing: Shamanism and Modern Medicine*, Boston and London 1985

Ader, Robert, (ed.), *Psychoneuroimmunology*, New York 1981

Bateson, Gregory, *Mind and Nature*, London, 1979

Bernal, J. D., *Science in History*, London, 1954

Bernheimer, Charles, and Kahane, Claire, *In Dora's Case: Freud – Hysteria – Feminism*, London 1985

Black, Stephen, *Mind and Body*, London, 1969

Blake, William, *Poetry and Prose* (ed. G. Keynes) Single volume edition, London, 1927

Bodley Scott, Ronald, *Cancer: The Facts*, Oxford, 1979

Boswell, James, *Everybody's Boswell* (with an abridgement of his *Life of Johnson*), London, 1930

Cannon, Walter, *The Wisdom of the Body*, New York, 1914

Capra, Fritjof, *The Turning Point*, London, 1982

Carter, James T., 'Health: As If We All Mattered', *Holistic Health Review*, Vol. 2, No. 2, (Spring) 1979 pp 6–9

Champion, R. H., 'Psoriasis', *British Medical Journal*, 1986, **292**, 1693

Cobb, L., *et al*, 'Evaluation of Internal Mammary Artery Ligation by Double-Blind Technic', *New England Journal of Medicine*, 260, 1959, pp 1115–18

Cooper, Cary L., (ed.) *Psychological Stress and Cancer*, London, 1984

Cornwell, Jocelyn, *Hard Earned Lives: Accounts of Health and Illness from East London*, London, 1984

Descartes, René, *Discourse on Method and other writings*, trans. F. E. Sutcliffe, London, 1968

Donne, John, *Complete Poetry and Selected Prose* ed. John Hayward, London, 1930

Douglas, Mary, *Purity and Danger*, London, 1970

Durdan-Smith, Jo, and De Simone, Diane, *Sex and the Brain*, London, 1983

Ellis, H. Havelock, *Studies in the Psychology of Sex*, (four volumes) New York, 1898

Entralgo, Pedro L., *Mind and Body: Psychosomatic Pathology, a Short History of the Evolution of Medical Thought*, London, 1955

Ewbank, Thomas, *A Descriptive and Historical Account of Hydraulic and Other Machines for Raising Water etc.*, London, 1842

Fest, Joachim, *Hitler*, London, 1977

Fisher, Richard B., *A Dictionary of Mental Health*, London, 1980

Freud, Sigmund, *The Psychopathology of Everyday Life*, (Pelican edition), London, 1938

Gardner, Martin (ed.), *The Annotated Alice*, London, 1965

Greer, Germaine, *The Female Eunuch*, London 1970

Greer, S., 'Psychological Response to Cancer', *The Lancet*, 13th October 1979, pp 785–7

Groddeck, George, *The Book of the It*, New York, 1949

Halsband, Robert, *The Life of Lady Mary Wortley Montague*, Oxford, 1956

Harrison, John, *Love Your Disease*, London, 1984

Hopkins, Gerard Manley, *The Journals and Papers* (ed. House, H. and Storey, G.) Oxford, 1966

Illich, Ivan, *Limits to Medicine*, London, 1977

Inglis, Brian, *The Diseases of Civilisation*, London, 1981

Insler, Vaclav and Lunenfeld, Bruno, *Infertility: Male and Female*, Edinburgh, 1986

Jones, Ernest, *The Life and Work of Sigmund Freud* (abridged edition) London, 1964

Jung, Carl Gustav, *Memories, Dreams, Reflections*, London, 1967

Kaptchuk, Ted and Croucher, Michael *The Healing Arts*, London, 1986

Karlins, Marvin, and Andrews, Lewis M., *Biofeedback*, London, 1975

Koestler, Arthur, *Bricks to Babel: Selected Writings with Comments by the Author*, London, 1980.

Leshan, Lawrence, *You Can Fight For Your Life*, London, 1984

Lewis, C. S., *A Grief Observed*, London, 1961

Lucas, Laddie, *Flying Colours*, London, 1985

McEvedy, C. P. and Beard, A. W., 'Concepts of Benign Encephalomy-elitis', *British Medical Journal*, 1970, 1, 11–15
McNeill, William, *Plagues and People*, London 1979
Marcus, Maria, *A Taste for Pain*, (trans. from the Danish by Joan Tate), London, 1981
Marcuse, F. L., *Hypnosis: Fact and Fiction*, London, 1959
Marnham, Patrick, *Lourdes: A Modern Pilgrimage*, London, 1980
Mason, A. A., *et al*, 'A Case of Congenital Ichthyoform Erythrodermia Treated by Hypnosis', *British Medical Journal*, 23rd August, 1952 pp 422–3
Maurois, André, *The Quest for Proust*, London, 1962
Medawar, Charles, *The Wrong Kind of Medicine*, London, 1984
Melzack, Ronald and Wall, Patrick, *The Challenge of Pain*, London, 1982
Miller, Jonathan, *The Body in Question*, London, 1978
Millett, Kate, *Sexual Politics*, London, 1971
Mitchell, Jeanette, *What is to be done about Health and Disease?*, London, 1984
Monod, Jacques, *Chance and Necessity*, London, 1974
Morovitz, Harold J., 'Rediscovering the Mind', *Psychology Today*, August 1980
Mulhallen, Jacqueline and Wright, D. J. M., 'Samuel Johnson: amateur physician', *Journal of the Royal Society of Medicine*, vol. 76, pp 217–222

Parish, J. Gordon, 'Epidemic Neuromyasthenia' in *Postgraduate Medical Journal*, November, 1978
Pfeffer, Naomi and Wollett, Ann, *The Experience of Infertility*, London, 1983
Plato, *The Timaeus* (trans. H. D. P. Lee) London, 1965
Powell, Anthony, *A Question of Upbringing*, London, 1951
Proust, Marcel, *Remembrance of Things Past* (trans. Scott Moncrieff and Terence Kilmartin), London, 1983

Reich, Wilhelm, *The Function of the Orgasm*, London, 1968
Rivers, William Halse, *Mind and Medicine*, London, 1920
Rose, Geoffrey and Marmot, M. G., 'Social Class and Coronary Heart Disease', *British Heart Journal*, 1981, 45, 13–19

Sacks, Oliver, *A Leg to Stand On*, London, 1986
Sacks, Oliver, *Awakenings*, (2nd edition), London, 1976
Sacks, Oliver, *Migraine* (revised edition), London, 1982
Schilder, Paul, *The Image and Appearance of the Human Body*, New York, 1964

Seville, R. H., 'Psoriasis and Stress I', *British Journal of Dermatology*, 1977, **97**, 297

Seville, R. H., 'Psoriasis and Stress II', *British Journal of Dermatology*, 1978, **98**, 151.

Seville, R. H., 'Psoriasis, Stress, Insight and Prognosis', *Seminars in Dermatology*, Vol. 2, no. 3, September, 1983

Seville, R. H. and Martin E., *Dermatological Nursing and Therapy*, Oxford, 1981

Shorter, Edward, *Bedside Manners: The Troubled History of Doctors and Patients*, London, 1986

Shorter, Edward, *A History of Women's Bodies*, London, 1984

Simeons, A. T. W., *Man's Presumptuous Brain*, London, 1960

Solzenitsyn, Alexander, *Cancer Ward* (trans. by Nicholas Bethell and David Burg, complete edition), London, 1970

Sontag, Susan, *Illness as Metaphor*, London, 1979

Suttie, Ian D., *The Origins of Love and Hate*, London, 1963

Taylor, Gordon Rattray, *A Natural History of Mind*, London, 1979

Thomas, Lewis, *The Youngest Science*, London, 1984

Trautmann, Bert, *Steppes To Wembley*, London, 1956

Tuchman, Barbara, *A Distant Mirror*, London, 1979

Tuke, Daniel Hack, *Illustrations of the Influence of the Mind upon the Body in Health and Disease, Designed to Elucidate the Action of the Imagination* (2nd edition), London, 1884

Updike, John, 'At War With My Skin', *New Yorker*, 2nd September, 1985

Updike, John, *Problems and Other Stories*, London, 1980

Veith, Ilse, *Hysteria: the History of a Disease*, Chicago, 1965

Walker, Benjamin, *Encyclopaedia of Metaphysical Medicine*, London, 1978

Walters, Allan, 'Psychogenic Regional Pain, *alias* Hysterical Pain', *Brain*, 1961, **84**, 1–18

Waxman, David, *Hypnosis; A Guide for Patients and Practitioners*, London, 1981

Williams, William Carlos, *Autobiography*, New York, 1967

Wingate, Peter, *The Penguin Medical Encyclopaedia*, (2nd edition), London, 1976

Winston, Robert, *Infertility: A Sympathetic Approach*, London, 1986

Wood, Clive, 'Good Behaviour for a Heart Attack', *New Scientist*, 13th March 1986, p 31

'Y', *Autobiography of an Englishman*, London, 1975

Index

243

All these books are available at your local bookshop or newsagent, or can be ordered direct from the publisher. Indicate the number of copies required and fill in the form below.

Send to: **CS Department, Pan Books Ltd., P.O. Box 40, Basingstoke, Hants.   RG21 2YT.**

or phone: 0256 469551 (Ansaphone), quoting title, author and Credit Card number.

Please enclose a remittance* to the value of the cover price plus: 60p for the first book plus 30p per copy for each additional book ordered to a maximum charge of £2.40 to cover postage and packing.

*Payment may be made in sterling by UK personal cheque, postal order, sterling draft or international money order, made payable to Pan Books Ltd.

Alternatively by Barclaycard/Access:

Card No.

Signature:

Applicable only in the UK and Republic of Ireland.

While every effort is made to keep prices low, it is sometimes necessary to increase prices at short notice. Pan Books reserve the right to show on covers and charge new retail prices which may differ from those advertised in the text or elsewhere.

NAME AND ADDRESS IN BLOCK LETTERS PLEASE:

....

Name————————————————————————

Address————————————————————————

————————————————————————————

————————————————————————————

3/87

ISC MEDICAL
Interview Skills Consulting

WB 110 ORG mcp

GP RECRUITMENT

7 DAY LOAN

Co

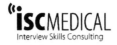

ISCMEDICAL
Interview Skills Consulting

Published by ISC Medical
Suite 434, Hamilton House, Mabledon Place, London WC1H 9BB
www.iscmedical.co.uk - Tel: 0845 226 9487

First edition: October 2007
Reprinted June 2008

ISBN13: 978-1-905812-11-0
A catalogue record of this book is available from the British Library.

Printed in the United Kingdom by:
Aidan's Ltd. Reg. Office 35 Ballards Lane, London N3 1XW